THE 6 PILLARS OF CHAKRA HEALING

89 Beginner Techniques & Hacks to Heal Your **Body, Mind, and Spirit**. Transform Your Life Through Energy Balancing. Guide to Practical Remedies for Health and Wellness

MONIQUE WAGNER

© **Copyright 2023 - All rights reserved.**

The content contained within this book may not be reproduced, duplicated or transmitted without direct written permission from the author or the publisher.

Under no circumstances will any blame or legal responsibility be held against the publisher, or author, for any damages, reparation, or monetary loss due to the information contained within this book, either directly or indirectly.

Legal Notice:

This book is copyright protected. It is only for personal use. You cannot amend, distribute, sell, use, quote or paraphrase any part, or the content within this book, without the consent of the author or publisher.

Disclaimer Notice:

Please note the information contained within this document is for educational and entertainment purposes only. All effort has been executed to present accurate, up to date, reliable, complete information. No warranties of any kind are declared or implied. Readers acknowledge that the author is not engaged in the rendering of legal, financial, medical or professional advice. The content within this book has been derived from various sources. Please consult a licensed professional before attempting any techniques outlined in this book.

By reading this document, the reader agrees that under no circumstances is the author responsible for any losses, direct or indirect, that are incurred as a result of the use of the information contained within this document, including, but not limited to, errors, omissions, or inaccuracies.

Table of Contents

Introduction 9

Pillar 1: Foundations 14

Chapter 1: Chakras Explained 17
What Are Chakras? 17
Crossover Practices 18
Common Misconceptions 20

Chapter 2: Origins and History 23
Where Are Chakras From? 24
Religious Origins 24
Chakra Timeline 27

Chapter 3: Energy 31
Prana 32
Nadi 32

Pillar 2: Systems 38

Chapter 4: Chakra Systems 41

What Are Chakra Systems? 42

What Is in a Chakra? 43

The Importance of Chakras in the Body 44

Chapter 5: Individual Chakras (Major) 47

Root Chakra 48

Sacral Chakra 49

Solar Plexus Chakra 50

Heart Chakra 51

Throat Chakra 52

Third Eye Chakra 54

Crown Chakra 55

Chapter 6: Higher Chakras 57

Earth Star Chakra 58

Soul Star Chakra 59

Universal Chakra 60

Galactic Chakra 60

Divine Chakra 61

Chapter 7: Individual Chakras (Minor) 63

The Foot Chakra 64

The Knee Chakra 65

The Pubic Chakra 65

Pillar 3: Relationships 68

Chapter 8: Chakras and the Endocrine System 71

What Is the Endocrine System? 72

Breakdown of the Chakra Connection 77

Chapter 9: Chakras and the Elements 79

What Are the Elements? 80

Earth 81

Water 84

Fire 86

Air 88

Ether 90

Light 91

Thought 91

Pillar 4: Activation 94

Chapter 10: Why Should You Open Your Chakras? 97

Target Issues in Your Life 98

Learn About Yourself 98

Enhance Other Spiritual Practices 99

Strengthen Mind-Body Connection 100

Chapter 11: How to Awaken Your Chakras 101

What Happens When Chakras Are Activated? 102

Where Do You Start? 102

Chakra by Chakra 103

Pillar 5: Balance 108

Chapter 12: What Is Chakra Balancing? 111

What Is the Difference Between Balancing and Activating? 112

How to Tell if Your Chakras Are Imbalanced 113

Chapter 13: How to Rebalance Your Chakras 119

Are Your Chakras Overactive or Underactive? 119

Chakra by Chakra 120

Pillar 6: Healing 126

Chapter 14: Practices 129

Ayurveda 130

Yoga 133

Meditation 135

Psychotherapy 136

Reiki 136

Chapter 15: Remedies 137

Allergies 137

Anger Management 138

Anxiety 138

Back Pain 138

Codependency 139

Confidence 139

Headaches 139

Joints 140

Sex 140

Trauma 141

Conclusion 143

Glossary 145

References 149

Introduction

The human body is a complex machine full of numerous systems and organs; it performs millions of actions a day, some conscious, some unconscious. In fact, the vast majority of tasks the human body performs are actually unconscious. Heartbeats, digestion, immune responses—all of these things happen without your conscious mind needing to be involved. Most people really have no idea what's going on inside their bodies at any given time. This is why people can live with a serious illness and not be aware of it or fight viruses while they are asleep. But there are more unconscious things going on inside the body than just basic health functions. Underneath all the physical processes of your body, there are also spiritual systems that underpin the very core of who you are, systems that work parallel to your body's physical functions but that are just as unconscious. Some people call it the soul, some the spirit self, but there is one system that categorizes this inner network according to parts of the body called chakras.

Chakras are an ancient South Asian philosophy that endeavors to explain these unseen systems that work throughout the human body. A lot of research has been done lately around the connection between the body and mental health. Many researchers are finding that there are great mental health benefits to things like exercise, healthy eating, and even gut bacteria. Western medicine is realizing more and more that there is a strong connection between the mind and the body and that all of our body systems are connected. Well, practitioners of chakra medicine have always known this. Chakras aim to explain and explore the complex ways in which our minds are linked to our bodies and how these links can be manipulated in order to ensure that all our faculties are working at their highest capacity.

So, what are chakras exactly? Well, chakras are essentially points identified in our bodies that have a certain significance. Each body part has a corresponding mental facet—an aspect of life or the self that is ruled by that particular body part. This is similar to how back pain is related to stress or how chronic fatigue is linked to digestive problems. Chakras attempt to define aspects of our bodies that are connected to aspects of our minds. The elements of life that chakras deal with, however, are often much deeper than Western medical science will really examine. For example, Western doctors will often talk about stress, grief, or trauma, but they won't talk about relationships, long-term goals, self-esteem, or spiritual identity. These things can be seen as a little too abstract or vague and sometimes are not even taken seriously at all by Western doctors. But chakra healers know that the bodily impacts of self-esteem can be just as powerful as those of trauma. In chakra healing, everything you feel has a reflection in the body and vice versa. By forging and recognizing this connection and explaining its intricacies, chakra healing aims to heal the mind through the body and the body through the mind.

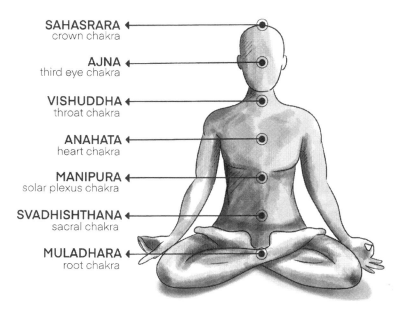

There are seven main chakras on the body which each correspond to a specific aspect of your life. The seven main chakras are the root chakra, the sacral chakra, the solar plexus chakra, the heart chakra, the throat chakra, the third eye chakra, and the crown chakra. Each of these seven has a corresponding body part, bodily system, set of possible ailments, and aspect of the self. In terms of physical assignment, this list goes from the bottom of your core, the tailbone, to the top of your head. The bottom, or root chakra, deals with the baser things in life, kind of like the bottom of the pyramid of needs. As you move up the body, you get to higher and higher purposes on the emotional chain, eventually culminating in the crown chakra, which deals with your spiritual self. Because of this scale, the chakras are often divided into two groups: the higher chakras and the lower chakras. Using this system of seven, you can categorize your body in terms of the ways it influences your mind.

So, how do chakras work exactly? Generally, chakra healers talk about chakras being "blocked" or "unblocked." When a chakra is blocked, you will usually see both psychological and physiological responses—a reflection in both your mental and physical health. For example, your throat chakra deals with not only your communication with others but also your general sinus, throat, and mouth area. So, if your throat chakra is blocked, you might find that you have sinus issues and feel like you aren't communicating very honestly or effectively with others. What chakra healing aims to do is help you identify which chakras on your body might be blocked and how you can go about unblocking them. Only by closely connecting the mind and the body can you really heal both.

In this book, we will give you a complete overview of chakra healing through six distinctive pillars. These pillars aim to divide chakra healing into six easy parts to help even the most inexperienced beginner become knowledgeable in the subject. In the first pillar, we will look at the foundations of chakra healing, explaining how they work and a little about their history. In the second pillar, we will dive deeper into the actual systems of the chakras, looking at each individual one and its role in your life. Then, in Pillar 3, we will branch out a little bit and look at the relationships that chakras have with other systems in your body as well as the world at large. After that, Pillar 4 will look at the ways in which you can activate your chakras, showing you more concrete and practical tips about fine-tuning your chakras. In Pillar 5, we will then talk about how to balance your chakras and ensure that they have strong relationships with one another. Finally, in Pillar 6, we will discuss the specific healing practices you can use with your chakras. Through these pillars, you will be able to see how understanding chakras and their applications can drastically improve your life and your connection with your body. You will also find 89 techniques, tips, and strategies to help you heal your body, mind, and spirit. These techniques, tips, and strategies are peppered throughout the entire book. And it's intentionally designed this way to serve as your guide along each step of the process. With this information, you will be able to live a more balanced and spiritual life.

Pillar 1:
Foundations

Chakras have been around for a great portion of human history. For millennia, they have helped people gain a more holistic understanding of their minds and bodies. This system helps us section off different facets of our lives to explain why we think and feel the way we do. For those who are seeking a stronger relationship with their bodies, chakras have served a very important purpose. In this pillar, we will start you on your chakra journey by outlining some of the key aspects of chakras. First, we will provide a general definition of chakras so that you are more aware of what they are and what they do. Then, we will talk about some of the common misconceptions associated with chakras. Following this, we will explain some of the origins of the practice, tracing its history from ancient times up to today. Finally, we will discuss chakras and their relationship with energy. By the end of this pillar, you will have a basic understanding of chakras to take forward into the rest of the book.

Chapter 1:
Chakras Explained

In the Introduction, we gave a vague description of the concept of chakras, describing them merely as "energy centers," but here we will get into the specifics of what chakras really are. In this chapter, we will be thoroughly defining the chakras and their meanings by listing the main ones and giving you a solid understanding of how they connect the mind and the body. We will also give you a list of common misconceptions surrounding chakras to help you recognize what chakras *aren't* as well as what they are.

What Are Chakras?

So, what are chakras exactly? What parts of the body do they encompass and how do they work? What is their purpose and how do they help us? Well, the word "chakra" in Sanskrit actually means "wheel." The individual chakra wheels are envisioned like discs on the spine. The seven chakras are then positioned as seven individual discs representing different spinal altitudes. Given the prevalence of the nervous system throughout the body and the importance of the spinal cord as the center of that system, it makes sense that this would be the center of the chakras as well. The idea of the chakras as wheels also speaks to their dynamic nature. Our chakras are all spinning, creating lively energy centers at these distinct points in our bodies. Essentially, chakras are seven energy-holding wheels marking specific points on our spinal cord.

Chakras are mainly described as being "balanced," "blocked," or "unblocked." When a certain chakra is blocked, it means that you will have problems in that particular part of your body, and this can also translate to having similar problems in the area of your life to which that chakra corresponds. Identifying the specific chakra in your body that is blocked can greatly help you to connect physical and psychological ailments. The process of chakra healing thus generally centers around unblocking or opening up your chakras. You can do this through energy healing, yoga, or many other practices, which we will discuss in more detail later in this book. When your chakras are opened up, you will have a stronger connection between your mind and body as well as relief in many of your systems. By harnessing the power of chakras, you can bring a strong sense of holistic health to your body and mind, clearing up many ailments that cannot be reached by any other kind of medicine.

Crossover Practices

There are many other spiritual healing practices that have a strong relationship to chakras. Many of these traditions evolved alongside one another, sharing philosophies and incorporating each other into their practices. They might also have characteristics that correspond to one another, encouraging you to combine certain ideas from one practice with its corresponding elements in the other one. Often, combining these practices with one another can help enhance each one individually. In this section, we will talk about some of the main spiritual practices that have crossover with chakras.

Crystals

Crystal healing is another important part of spiritual practice. Crystals that come from the ground have strong vibrational powers which can preside over certain aspects of life and the body, similar to chakras. Most crystals have a corresponding chakra with which they connect strongly. Many people will incorporate crystals into their chakra healing, and vice versa, using corresponding crystals to help heal specific chakras.

Astrology

Another spiritual practice that corresponds with chakras is astrology, particularly the planets. In ancient astronomy, there were seven planetary bodies: the sun, the moon, Mercury, Venus, Mars, Jupiter, and Saturn. The outer planets had not been discovered yet, so ancient astrology operated on a system of seven. If you notice, there are also seven chakras, which is no coincidence. Each chakra is associated with a different planet. The root chakra is associated with Mars, the sacral chakra with Mercury, the solar plexus chakra with Jupiter, the heart chakra with Venus, the throat chakra with Saturn, the third eye chakra with the sun, and the crown chakra with the moon. Each of these chakras also corresponds with those planets' associated qualities in astrology. On your birth chart, you will be able to see the position of all your planets within the zodiac. For example, your Mercury might be in Gemini or your Mars in Sagittarius. When looking at your birth chart, consider how some of these planetary positions might relate to your chakra system.

Yoga

Yoga is probably the spiritual practice that is most closely related to chakras. Yoga evolved alongside chakras and is inextricably linked to chakra philosophy. Like chakras, yoga is a practice that aims to connect the mind and the body, incorporating both physical movement and mindfulness in order to create this connection. Many yoga poses and sequences are based on certain chakras or chakra systems. In the practice of chakra healing, yoga is often used extensively to help unblock certain chakras. Yoga promotes balance in the body, building strength, and always returns to the core, or the spinal cord. It helps you to balance your chakras and unblock certain ones that might be closed. In other words, you will need to know at least a little bit about yoga in order to practice chakras, and vice versa!

Common Misconceptions

As with any spiritual practice, there are a lot of misconceptions people have about chakras. How many people have told you that astrology is "nonsense" because everyone born in June can't possibly have the same personality? Or that crystals are just rocks that may offer a placebo effect? Skeptics and misinterpreters are a source of aggravation for many spiritual healers. People who don't understand the nuances of a particular spiritual system can be extremely frustrating. The same goes for chakras. Here, we will look at some of the most common misconceptions people tend to have about chakra healing.

Misconception #1: There Is Only One Chakra System

Because of how old and widespread the concept of chakras is, there are a lot of different systems people have practiced over the years. The system that we are discussing in this book is just one of many that have evolved over time. Because chakras are so fluid as a system, there are many ways to practice them, and no one way is necessarily right or wrong. If you get very into chakras, you can try different practices for yourself. However, it is never advisable to mix practices with one another. This will result in unsatisfying results and create a mixed relationship with your chakras. So, no matter the practice you choose to follow, make sure that you are consistent about it.

Misconception #2: The Chakras Exist in Physical Space

Although we did talk about how the chakras are located in specific areas of the body, they are not actually physically located in your body. Likewise, they do not necessarily physically resemble or associate with the qualities we ascribe to them, such as colors. Instead, they are focal points for visualization. They help us to see past the simple biological functions of the body and into the more minute functions of the visualizing mind. Thus, it is not very helpful to think of your chakras as a physical reality like your actual spinal cord. Instead, think of your chakras as focal points, parts of your body that need attention, not literal discs spinning around your spinal cord.

Misconception #3: There Are Only Seven Chakras

As we said above, there are many different chakra systems in the world. Some involve the seven-chakra system, which is the one we are focusing on in this book. However, there are many systems that include different numbers of chakras—anywhere from five to hundreds. You can think of the differences in the number of chakras as some systems involving more focus and attention rather than other systems leaving things out. Systems with fewer chakras tend to condense ideas into larger sections, whereas systems with more chakras tend to split the body into smaller parts that preside over more specific areas. Thus, when you are choosing a chakra system, reflect on the level of specificity you want.

Chapter 2:
Origins and History

Chakras did not come out of nowhere! Moreover, the ways we practice chakra healing today, especially in the Western world, did not come out of nowhere either. Current chakra practice is the result of a long history that spans the whole world. Those who know a lot about chakras will tell you that there is a lot more to them than meets the eye and that it took us a long time to get to where we are today. In this chapter, we will be looking at some of the most essential aspects of chakra origins. We will first be looking at the geographic origins, tracing the places that made chakras what they are today. Then, we will be looking at the timeline of the history of chakras, telling the story from their earliest origins through their maintenance over the course of history up until the current chakra practices of today. By the end of this chapter, you will be well-versed in where chakras came from and how they've changed over time, giving you a clearer picture of how their current practice came to be.

Where Are Chakras From?

Chakras have spread far and wide throughout the world today. In almost every country on Earth, you will find someone who practices chakra healing. Most people around the world have heard of chakras, and there are countless people across borders and cultures who have brought a version of chakra practice into their spiritual healing journeys. But it wasn't always this way. In fact, chakras actually have very specific origins in the Indian subcontinent, known today as South Asia, or the collection of countries of India, Sri Lanka, Bangladesh, and Pakistan. In this part of the world, we can trace the origins of chakras. To this day, chakras are still practiced widely throughout South Asia and are very commonly associated with other aspects of South Asian culture and spiritual practices. Often, dedicated chakra healers will make pilgrimages to parts of India to try and trace the geographical roots of the practice that has brought so much joy and healing to their lives.

Religious Origins

A discussion of chakra healing would not be complete without a discussion of the religions with which chakras are associated. There are two main religions with origins in South Asia: Hinduism and Buddhism. Both of these religions have strong relationships with chakras and warrant a thorough discussion of the ways they have incorporated chakras into their practices throughout history. In this section, we will discuss how chakras fit into Hinduism and Buddhism in both historical and contemporary practice.

Hinduism

Chakras are inherently a Hindu concept. Hinduism is one of the oldest widely practiced religions in the world. It has its origins in Ancient India, dating back thousands of years. The beginnings of Hinduism are all contained within certain Sanskrit texts called the "Vedas." These are a dense collection of texts that detail the main philosophies of the Hindu religion. They are a compilation of many different documents throughout history, so it is difficult to date their origins. Chakras have their roots in these documents and thus can be said to be at least a few thousand years old. Evolving alongside the Hindu tradition, chakras also have Hindi names along with their English names. So, the root chakra is the *muladhara*, the sacral chakra is the *swadhisthana*, the solar plexus chakra is the *manipura*, the heart chakra is the *anahata*, the throat chakra is the *vishuddha*, the third eye chakra is the *ajna*, and the crown chakra is the *sahasrara*. For the purposes of this book, we will be using their English names, but it's important to remember that they were originally used in Hindu practice.

Chakras are linked to many different Hindu practices and are still used in the contemporary Hindu religion. The way chakras work in this practice is through the passing of knowledge from the bottom to the top. The chakra energy is believed to be sacred and to come from above from the highest form of life known as Brahman. Naturally, these energies tend to pool around our root chakra, concentrating in the lowest part of our bodies. With meditation and yoga, the goal is to raise these energies through the chakras. As this energy moves up the chain of the body, we become more attentive to higher knowledge and gain a more enlightened view of life and the universe. The crown chakra is the ultimate goal of this practice, concentrating our energies in the highest place on our spiritual body to become aware of things beyond the visible universe and to gain deeper insight.

Besides yoga and meditation, another aspect of Hinduism that relates to the chakras is the gods themselves. As you might already know, Hinduism is a polytheistic religion, which means that they worship more than one god. Unlike Christianity or Islam, which have one central spiritual being, Hinduism has many different gods that all relate to different ideas or facets of life. This is similar to the Greek gods, such as Aphrodite and Dionysus, who preside over love and wine respectively, or even the patron saint system of Catholicism, which assigns different areas to different saints. Consequently, all the gods in Hindu theology have their own unique role to play in the cosmic system. And, as you might have guessed, they each have a chakra that they are associated with. The root chakra is associated with Ganesh, the god of beginnings who takes the form of an elephant; the sacral chakra is associated with Vishnu, the god of preservation and benevolence; the solar plexus chakra is associated with Siva, the god of destruction and renewal; the heart chakra is associated with Ishvara, a more conceptual god who is a center of spiritual enlightenment; the throat chakra is associated with Sadasiva, the highest form of Siva representing fulfillment and longevity; the third eye chakra is associated with Ardhanarishvara, the composite of Siva and his consort Parvati representing the harmony between male and female; and finally the crown chakra is associated with Lord Siva, or the highest form of Siva. When you focus on a particular chakra in Hindu theology, you are also channeling or asking for help from a particular god in the pantheon.

Buddhism

Compared to Hinduism, Buddhism is actually a relatively new religion, though it still has origins in ancient times. Buddhism started around 500 B.C.E. in what is now the northern region of the nation of India. It began with a prince named Siddhartha who chose to leave his aristocratic existence to achieve a more collective understanding of reality through charity and living among the poor. Buddhist teachings thus purport that there is no true boundary between people, nor between humans and animals, and therefore selflessness is the only true expression of reality. From there, Buddhism spread throughout the subcontinent and into parts of Asia such as China, Korea, and Japan, where it continues to be very widely practiced today.

Buddhism is very different from Hinduism, but because Buddhism began in South Asia as well, there are many Hindu concepts that were carried over to it. Though there are technically no mentions of chakras in the original Buddhist texts, there are prevalent ideas that can be seen to have origins in Hindu chakra practice. Buddhist use of the chakras is found most prominently in Tibetan Buddhism, which is a particular sect of Buddhism that has carried over many Hindu aspects to Buddhist theology. In Tibetan Buddhism, there is a strong tradition of chakra meditation similar to that in Hinduism. However, there are also other Buddhist systems that use chakra or energy exercises. For example, Chinese or Zen Buddhism acknowledges three main chakras: the lower *dantian* (similar to the solar plexus or sacral), the middle *dantian* (similar to the heart or throat), and the upper *dantian* (similar to the third eye or crown). In this chakra practice, we can see the roots of Hindu chakras. So, while chakras aren't as embedded in Buddhist theology as they are in Hindu theology, there are still aspects of chakra healing found within Buddhism.

Chakra Timeline

Now that you are familiar with the religious origins of chakras, we can talk a bit about how chakras have evolved throughout history. As we said earlier in this chapter, they do have their roots in the present-day country of India, but they have been found to spread far outside its borders, influencing many other cultures and spiritual movements over the course of history. In this section, we will give you a brief overview of the evolution of chakra practice.

Ancient Period

As we discussed in the religion section of this chapter, chakras are ancient in origin. They find their roots in texts thousands of years old and are thus one of the oldest continuously practiced traditions. In the ancient period, chakras were fairly confined to Hindu communities and kingdoms. They formed a significant component of Hindu practice and were also used in healing. Many different regions throughout South Asia practiced a version of chakras, some being different from others. At that time, things like the number of chakras, their exact meanings, and their relationships with things like colors were not yet fixed. Communities in different areas believed in different numbers of chakras and ascribed different meanings to them. At that time, there was not the same seven-chakra system we have today, especially not in relation to specific psychological states. This system was still in flux, made unique by every region that put its own spin on the practice.

Middle Ages

During the Middle Ages, the most important thing to happen throughout Afro-Eurasia was the rise of Islam. As the religion took off in the Middle East, it began to spread outward, both west into Europe and North Africa as well as east toward South Asia. The northern region of modern-day India, which you will remember was the place of origin for Buddhism, was colonized by a Muslim empire known as the Mughals. The Mughal Empire was extremely powerful in this region and lasted from the early 1500s to the late 1800s. Much of contemporary Indian culture and architecture has its origins in this period, including the iconic Taj Mahal itself. The wealth and influence of this empire were staggering, meaning that much of the subcontinent was Muslim for a time. Because Islam is a monotheistic religion that is more focused on scholarship and prayer than meditation and yoga, chakra practices were not as common during this time. However, there were still many autonomous Hindu regions that continued to practice chakras as before. But once the Mughals were no more, an even greater force was coming for India that would have another massive effect on their religious identity: the British.

Modern Revival

Starting in the 1500s, or the "Age of Exploration," Europeans began to grow dependent upon an economic system based on conquest and trade, resulting in a colonial hold over a large portion of the world. Alongside this age of colonialism, a new movement sprang up in French and English philosophy called "Orientalism," starting around the 1700s–1800s. During this period, many French and British scholars became fascinated by "Eastern" religions and philosophies as well as art and decor. Many would travel to places like China and South Asia to learn about religious practices and to purchase decorative items. While these French philosophers were furnishing their houses with Chinese pottery and Indian textiles, they were also furnishing their minds with these new ideas. Orientalism as a concept eventually gave way to many New Age movements that sought to incorporate elements of Eastern religions like Hinduism and Buddhism into their lives. One of the concepts that they incorporated was chakras. Throughout the 19th and 20th centuries, chakras gradually became more and more popular in the West. This coincided with movements like spiritualism, occultism, and New Age philosophy. It is here that we truly see the rise of the seven-chakra system and the contemporary Western chakra system in general.

Chapter 3:
Energy

Moving on to a more in-depth understanding of the chakras, we are now ready to talk about the specificities of the chakra system. One of the most important concepts in chakra practice is energy. We have already mentioned energy as a concept thus far, but only vaguely. You might think of energy as simply the opposite of fatigue. This is how we typically use the word in the Western world. We say, "I have no energy," when we really mean we are tired or feel that our bodies don't have enough fuel to function. However, from a spiritual standpoint, this would always be a false statement. You always have energy flowing through you, no matter how tired you feel. More than that, in certain spiritual systems, you have many different kinds of energy that all relate to one another in different ways. Systems like the chakra framework can help you to understand the different kinds of energies within you and to harness these energies and nurture them so that they can work properly. Chakra practice in particular has a very specific relationship with the concept of energy. In this chapter, we will talk about the precise ways in which chakra practice describes and categorizes energy.

Prana

Many different religions and practices have a specific word to mean "energy," and chakra practice is no different. In this particular philosophy, energy is known as "prana." Prana is a way of describing the life force within all of us, much like the concept of "Chi" in Chinese philosophy. Prana is present in all things on earth, including things that might seem to be inanimate, which means that humans, animals, plants, and rocks alike have prana at their core. This is a guiding concept in the world of crystal healing which operates on the idea that rocks and minerals have an essential energy to them that can be used for healing purposes. Some people also believe that prana is a vital principle in life. There is an element of oneness to prana that connects all the living things that have it at their center. It helps us to see and connect with the vital life force at the core of our beings as well as the core beings of others. We can see how this Hindu concept influenced the core life force aspect of Buddhist theology, connecting all things on Earth with a common thread. However, there is still more to prana than just a central life force; it is also channeled through pathways known as "nadi."

Nadi

The division of prana is done by nadi, which shape prana into the form it needs to take in order to successfully create life force. The nadi are actually very similar to the chakra system itself, sectioning off the body into different parts that are defined by certain characteristics and functions. However, unlike chakras, which run from the bottom of the body to the top, nadi run from side to side. These intersect with the chakras in very interesting ways and can change or add nuance to the existing meanings of the chakras. If you don't consider your nadi, then you might be getting an incomplete version of your chakra readings. This is very similar to astrology, which has multiple different signs that interact with each other. Knowing your main sign, or sun sign, can be useful and tell you a lot about yourself, but if you aren't aware of your moon sign, rising sign, planets, or houses, then you will always have an incomplete picture of your astrological identity. The same goes for chakras. Think of the nadi as your moon sign, another facet of the chakra system that can help you further expand your knowledge of the chakras in your body. Now, just like with chakras, there are actually many different nadi systems that identify different numbers of nadi in the body. Some identify three, some fourteen, and some many more. Each of these systems will have a varying degree of complexity based on the number of nadi it identifies. However, for the purposes of this book, we will be looking at three of the most important nadi. In this section, we will list these three for you and explain their significance within the body.

Ida Nadi

First off, we have the ida nadi, which is located on the left side of the body. Some people call this the "negative" side of the body, or your negative nadi. However, negative doesn't necessarily have a, well, negative connotation in this context. Oftentimes in spirituality, negativity doesn't mean bad or malicious but merely one side of a duality. Thus, you can think of "negative" things in spirituality with a more neutral connotation, meaning simply the inverse of a positive thing. Imagine them as the negative numbers on a number line, running parallel to the positive numbers but in the opposite direction. You can also think of them as the negative side of a battery or the south pole of a magnet. You can even think of them like negative space in a painting or a photograph, not full of dynamism, but a necessary aspect of the composition which gives the piece clarity and freshness. So, there is no need to avoid or look away from your ida nadi, even though it is categorized as technically negative.

The nadi are essentially categorized according to dualities, so the ida nadi will be everything the pingala, its corresponding nadi, is not. Ida is often associated with feminine energy. We can see in many other spiritual dualities that feminine energy is commonly associated with the moon, coolness, and emotions. The elements of earth and water are also associated with the ida nadi. Many female goddesses throughout the world are also associated with these things, such as the Greek goddess Artemis, who presides over the moon. Other aspects of ida nadi are creativity and inspiration as well as introversion. Think of the stereotypical "reserved genius," and you will have some idea about the central philosophy of the nadi. One interesting aspect of the nadi is that they recognize one fundamental concept in brain science, which is that the left side of the brain actually controls the right side of the body and vice versa. Therefore, you might have been confused about this nadi, since we typically think of the right brain as the creative side and the left side as the logical side. Well, don't worry because this is actually true of the nadi. Ida might preside over the left side of the body, but it presides over the right side of the brain as well. Ida also connects with the nervous system of the body and thus controls much of your body's physical functions, being the inherent link between the brain and the body. For this reason, it is a central aspect of your body and mind.

One of the most common misconceptions about the ida nadi, and the nadi in general, is that only women can really connect with it. Because it is associated with feminine energy, male chakra practitioners might be reluctant to lean into it. However, this is a much too literal interpretation of the concept of the ida nadi. Just as negative energy does not mean bad energy, feminine energy does not necessarily mean biologically or literally female. Basically, you can be any gender and associate strongly with your ida nadi. If you want to get in touch with your feminine side or bring some free-flowing energy into your chakra practice, you should try to channel your energy through this side of your body, allowing your prana to flow properly and release its powers.

Pingala Nadi

In contrast to the ida nadi is the pingala nadi. This nadi is associated with masculine energy and is the mirror image of ida nadi in every way. It is located on the right side of the body but controls the left side of the brain. As you might expect, it is associated with the sun, meaning that it is the warm, enlightening force to the ida's shadowy, cool force. The pingala nadi also leans more heavily into logic and reason. Elements like fire and air are also associated with the pingala nadi. We can see these associations in other religions as well. For example, the Greek god Apollo is Artemis's twin brother and is associated with the sun, while the hypermasculine god Ares is associated with fire and vigor. These associations are baked deeply into many religious systems from around the world, and thus it is highly important to recognize them in tandem with one another. Again, you don't have to be male to connect with your pingala nadi. Anyone can focus on this force in their life. It can help you realize some of the deeper ideas formed in the ida and put them into motion. Channeling your pingala nadi will help you bring things into action and create dynamism throughout your life.

Sushumna Nadi

So, you might be wondering, if the former two nadi are mirror images of each other, how can there be a third nadi? Well, the third nadi is actually located directly in the middle of the spine and represents the merging of the two. This nadi is the most important as it represents an existence free of dualities and contradictions. Only by truly balancing and awakening your ida and pingala nadi can you come to activate your sushumna nadi. This highlights the importance of your ida and pingala nadi as collaborators rather than enemies. You should not think of them as two sides of a chessboard but rather as two sides of a married couple. Separated and working independently, these nadi will only have themselves to rely on, working only with the tools they have within their own realms, but together, they can combine their energies to become greater than the sum of their parts. All the deep ideas forged in your ida nadi can finally be freed and come to fruition in your pingala nadi, and all the energy found in your pingala nadi can be used to nurture and care for others using your ida nadi. This is very similar to the concept of yin and yang, which also constructs opposing forces that strongly influence one another and need to be merged in order to truly reach enlightenment. Unfortunately, most people do not find the strength to connect these two nadi in order to fundamentally awaken their sushumna nadi and thus spend their lives with two divided halves. In order to truly create harmony in your body, you must learn through chakra healing to merge these energies to create a balanced whole.

Pillar 2: Systems

In Pillar 1, we discussed all of the basic information associated with chakras. We let you know how the chakras work and where they came from. By now, you should be starting to get a firmer grip on the working world of chakras. In this section, we will be moving into a more detailed understanding of the chakras. First, in Chapter 4, we will discuss the chakras as a system, illustrating how they work in tandem with one another to form a harmonious whole. Next, in Chapter 5, we will give you a thorough explanation of the individual major chakras themselves. These are the seven chakras we have already talked about that form the basis for the Western chakras. Then, in Chapter 6, we will talk about the higher chakras, which is a separate system made up of five different chakras that exist on a different plane from the major chakras. Finally, in Chapter 7, we will discuss the minor or lower chakras, which center around smaller, more specific sections of the body. In these chapters, you will get a stronger sense of the main chakras themselves as well as more context around how they function in relation to other chakra systems.

Chapter 4:
Chakra Systems

The chakras are not forces that act in and of themselves. We have touched a little on the individual meanings of the chakras thus far in the book, but it is important to take a step back and assert that the main aspect of chakras is their connection to one another and their flow throughout the body. As we have seen with the nadi, the ability to truly merge and connect your chakras with one another is a central aspect of how they operate within the body. Only by treating your chakras as a single unified system can you come to understand them and their flow. You cannot fix one without the others being finely tuned. You can think of your chakra systems just like ingredients in a recipe. Has it ever happened that you had all the right ingredients for a recipe, all of excellent quality, but you mixed them together in the wrong order and the recipe completely fell flat? Well, that's how you have to think about chakras. Even if you balance or unblock them all individually, you will only be able to truly heal them if you think of them as a single system that needs to be balanced. In this chapter, we will discuss how the chakra system treats itself as a system of balance and harmony.

What Are Chakra Systems?

So, first of all, what are chakra systems and how do they work? How do these distinctive areas of the body connect to one another? Well, the chakra system all goes back to the discussion we had in Chapter 2 about the Hindu origins of chakras. In this philosophy, chakras are not distinctive aspects of your body at all but a network of areas that channel energy through them. You can think of this system as being multiple floors in an office building with the spine as an elevator connecting them all. The bottom floors are basic functions like electricity, bathrooms, power sources, and of course, the foundation of the building itself. Then, as you move to the middle floors, you get administration and communication departments, which manage the functions of the company and connect it to the outside world. On the top floors of the building are the executives, the creative teams, and the CEO, all of whom deal with the highest functions of the company, planning its future and coming up with groundbreaking ideas that will take it far. As you can see, all of these areas work independently, but they have clear relationships with one another and a movement from top to bottom. If you center yourself too much on your bottom floors, or lower chakras, then you will never gain higher knowledge or foresight. But conversely, if you neglect these foundational chakras, or basic company functions, the rest of the building will suffer. From this analogy, we can see how the energy flow throughout the chakras is crucial for their spiritual function. Using meditation and yoga to facilitate the spread of this energy, especially from the bottom to the top, is a central part of chakra practice and philosophy.

What Is in a Chakra?

There has been a lot of discussion in modern Western culture about the body's role in psychological states. Books like Bessel van der Kolk's *The Body Keeps the Score* detail how many of our experiences, both good and bad, can be stored in the body's organs and nervous system (2014). You can even see this playing out in real time with physical anxiety symptoms or physical triggers associated with trauma. According to chakra theory and practice, the body really does keep the score. For millennia, chakra healers have asserted that chakras not only store energy centers but also core aspects of our lives, both mental and physical. Chakras can keep track of your memories, your experiences, and your habits. They have a keen memory and serve as a way to create who we are. But as you probably know, the things that make you who you are can also be the things that limit you. Understanding your chakras and what they are storing inside them is integral to forming a more complete understanding of yourself and where you have come from.

Chakras can store even more than the past; they can also store the future. The state your chakras are in determines what your future self or life will look like. Furthermore, your chakras also hold your dreams, goals, and beliefs about the future. We see this more literally played out in the higher chakras, which deal with foresight and planning, but also in the lower chakras which deal with identity and self-esteem. The beliefs you have about yourself and your future are stored deep within your chakras, meaning that your chakras have an important influence on your future. Thus, with this future influence, we can see how chakra energy flows freely between the body and the outside world. Just as chakras are influenced by your ideas and experiences, so too are your future experiences influenced by your chakras. From this, you can really see how the body creates reality and how reality creates the body. Use this knowledge to feel a stronger connection to the world around you.

The Importance of Chakras in the Body

So, now that you know how connected the chakras really are, you can begin to see how a blockage in any of your chakras can really affect your ability to function. One chakra being blocked does not just mean that the certain aspect of your life controlled by that chakra is blocked but also that energy cannot freely flow throughout your whole system. You can think of this like a drain being blocked. Water can flow above and below the block but not through it, so your drain is unusable simply because one small part of it is not functioning properly. For a more complex analogy, we can turn back to our seven-floor office building. Let's say floor five is the communications department, representing the throat chakra. If this department stops working properly, the other departments might not be affected right away as they are still going about their business. But slowly, the company's relationships with other firms will deteriorate, beginning to erode their capacity for outreach. They will lose advertisements, which will lead to fewer new clients, and eventually reduced profits. They will also not be able to respond to customer complaints, which might lead to losing even repeat customers who were previously loyal. All of these repercussions will eventually lead to cuts in other departments, and if not fixed, a complete shutdown of the company. As you can see, just removing one essential aspect of the function of the company can lead to a massive restructuring and possibly even bankruptcy.

Let's map this back onto a human being and their chakra identity. If you have a blockage in your throat chakra, you might struggle with communication, be dishonest, or have social anxiety. These kinds of things won't necessarily directly affect your other chakras and their functions, since they will be operating on different wavelengths. However, over time, the struggles you are facing because of your throat chakra block will eventually come to affect the other facets of your life. Struggling with communication can ruin relationships, which touches your heart chakra. Being dishonest hurts your social reputation, which can affect your self-esteem and relationships. Having social anxiety can mean you withdraw from the world, even your friends and family, which disrupts your sense of home and self, affecting your root chakra. All of these reverberations will eventually block your ability to flow energy up to your crown chakra and truly have foresight in the world. What you will be left with is a mind preoccupied with the petty issues of the everyday and the inability to truly seek enlightened thought.

Chapter 5:
Individual Chakras (Major)

Understanding the role the chakras play in each others' function is extremely important, but just as important is understanding how they work individually. Only by deeply exploring each chakra can you begin to recognize which ones you might have blocked and learn how to go about unblocking them. This will help you identify areas in your life that you feel might be affected by the chakra blockages and create a stronger sense of who you are. In this chapter, we will talk in-depth about each of the individual major chakras by giving you core information about the facets of life each one presides over as well as additional information about them and associations they might have.

Root Chakra

Associated Color:

Red

Associated Element:

Earth

Associated Body Parts:

The base of the spine, also known as the pelvic floor, where the earth and the body make contact

Description

The root chakra is the base of the whole chakra system. This means that it exists in a duality. On one hand, it deals with the baser aspects of human life, meaning that it is the least important chakra. But on the other hand, it is also the root of many aspects of your sense of self, including your core identity, your origins, and your connection to your bodily functions. It forms a large part of both your everyday living and your unconscious mind. Some people even think of the root chakra as representing a more animalistic side of human nature, showing us the basest of our instincts. However, this is one of the worst chakras to have unbalanced. Since energy tends to be concentrated here, with the goal of moving up toward the crown chakra, having a blocked root chakra means that your energy can't even move up to the next chakra, the sacral chakra. If your root chakra is unbalanced, then there is a very strong likelihood that your whole chakra system in general is badly unbalanced and lacks any flow whatsoever. Your higher chakras will be cut off from their energy source, and you will be left feeling like you have neither roots nor wisdom. Making sure this chakra is open and flowing freely is essential to the function of the entire chakra system.

Sacral Chakra

Associated Color:

Orange

Associated Element:

Water

Associated Body Parts:

The lower abdomen or genitals

Description

The sacral chakra is the center of your desire function. Thus, it presides over both sexuality and creative drive. It is the area in which many of your core ideas form. You need this chakra to give you a kind of life force. If your root chakra is your connection to the earth, then your sacral chakra is the drive that allows you to soar from it. Another big part of your sacral chakra is self-esteem. This relates not to the general self-esteem we might associate with the social world but to a deeper inner self-esteem that relates to our most intimate selves. This is a side of our personality that we might only share with ourselves or our intimate partners. When this self-esteem is threatened, it is much more serious than just being embarrassed—it is crushing to our sense of self. Thus, the sacral chakra represents another facet of our foundation of self, this time relating to our abilities more than our origins.

When your sacral chakra is unbalanced, you might very well react with frustration or anger. This can either be directed at yourself or others, but it stems from deep feelings of inadequacy. A blocked sacral chakra might find you failing to live up to your own expectations, which can result in you feeling frustrated with your situation and lashing out. You might also experience blocks both creatively and sexually. Creatively, this can look like writer's block or even just a lack of energy to complete the creative tasks you want to complete. Sexually, it can either come in the form of aversion or repression, or it can go in the other direction toward sexual obsession. Sometimes, this symptom can be physical, leading to sexual dysfunction or bladder issues. However, when this chakra is well-balanced, then you will feel a strong sense of accomplishment and pride in your achievements. You will also have the inner confidence to trust your own intuition and feelings.

Solar Plexus Chakra

Associated Color:

Yellow

Associated Element:

Fire

Associated Body Parts:

The stomach area or upper abdomen

Description

Your solar plexus chakra is where the ego tends to come in. As we move upward through the body's chakras, we start to get into the more social aspects of the world. Because it is still in the lower half of the chakras, the solar plexus chakra deals with the view of the self as it pertains to others. This is similar to the self-esteem-based sacral chakra but takes a particular focus on relationships with others. Your solar plexus chakra is thus connected more to your general acceptance by society or your friends rather than your evaluation of your own abilities. Things like popularity, social standing, and even just generally feeling loved by people can influence the self-esteem related to your solar plexus chakra.

When your solar plexus chakra becomes blocked, you will likely struggle to feel relevant in the world. You might feel isolated, unloved, unattractive, or useless. These feelings are directly related to a damaged ego, which feels like it is not performing for others in the way it wants to. Because the physical stomach is such a delicate organ, this is also an area with a lot of room for physical symptoms. A blocked solar plexus chakra can lead to a host of digestive problems, including food sensitivities and a tendency to throw up easily. However, if you gain the ability to balance it properly, then you will be able to face the world with more confidence and focus.

Heart Chakra

Associated Color:

Green

Associated Element:

Air

Associated Body Parts:

The chest

Description

It's easy to guess the heart chakra's purpose: love, compassion, and connection with others. As the center chakra on the body, it deals with neither personal nor outward-looking self-esteem but instead equally balances the two. This chakra is the connecting force between you and others, thus constructing an important link between the upper and lower chakras.

Your heart chakra presides over everything regarding your relationships, helping you to empathize with others, understand their needs, and communicate your own needs to them. In other words, it weighs yourself and others equally, striving to create strong two-way relationships in your life.

An unbalanced heart chakra can lead to many difficulties in your relationships. This will often take the form of hostility toward others. Negative feelings about other people, such as jealousy and anger, will usually be the manifestation. You might find yourself lashing out at loved ones or expecting the worst of people even though they haven't done anything wrong. Another common way your unbalanced heart chakra might manifest is through trust issues. You might find your attachment style turns anxious, leading you to struggle to keep your relationships close. You might also experience physical symptoms like chest pain or heartburn from an unbalanced heart chakra. Someone whose heart chakra is well-balanced will be open to others, ready to give and receive love, and feel genuinely part of a strong community. This is the ideal state to be in and helps you build intimate relationships and feel truly fulfilled.

Throat Chakra

Associated Color:

Blue

Associated Element:

Space

Associated Body Parts:

The throat as well as the neck area and sinuses

Description

The throat chakra is particularly concerned with the workings of the voice box, especially metaphorically speaking. The throat chakra presides over all things relating to your communication and vocal qualities. The way you speak and what you choose to use your words for are strongly influenced by the throat chakra. Consequently, it is also focused on a more public version of the interpersonal heart chakra. While the heart chakra focuses on your strong bonds with the important people in your life, the throat chakra focuses more on the public relationships in your broader life, looking further outward to things such as how you conduct yourself in the public sphere and how you convey your ideas to others. Being the communication chakra, the throat chakra deals with the wider social world and your ability to share yourself with it.

If your throat chakra is unbalanced, your communication and self-expression skills will suffer greatly. There are two ways this can go. The first way is that you become an incredibly timid person who struggles to express yourself. You might become socially reclusive or shy away from things like public speaking or performing in any way. This creates a very insular person who might have an excellent inner life but who struggles to bring that out into the greater world. The second way it can go is that you become a manipulative person who is confident in your social abilities but uses them for bad instead of good. You might be dishonest, prone to gossip, and possibly even outright cruel to people's faces. Both of these outcomes are not desirable and result in a person who struggles to have a healthy relationship with the outside world. Physical symptoms might also ensue; illnesses such as frequent head colds, sore throats, enlarged tonsils, and sinus infections are all related to a blocked throat chakra. When you finally manage to balance your throat chakra, you will be able to enjoy healthy and honest communication with others and be able to project yourself as a trustworthy and articulate person.

Third Eye Chakra

Associated Color:

Indigo

Associated Element:

No associated element

Associated Body Parts:

Between the eyes

Description

The third eye chakra is the second-highest chakra in the system and is where we first reach an area that is beyond everyday human life. The "third eye" is a commonly used term in the West, usually used to describe someone "opening their third eye" in order to see a higher reality. In chakra healing, the third eye is somewhat related to this concept, but it is more related to knowledge of the self and intuition. Essentially, when you use your third eye, you are stepping outside of your life and seeing it from a more objective standpoint. This allows you to get some distance from situations you might have grown too accustomed to and are thus struggling to see past. It will help you make long-term plans for your life and sort out what values are really and truly important to you. At the same time, the third eye chakra is also about connecting more strongly with your intuition and feeling more present in yourself or your body. So, it is simultaneously about intuition and greater objectivity.

When your third eye chakra is blocked, you will be very shortsighted in the way you think about and plan your life. Some might say this state is like not being able to see the forest for the trees—you cannot see your life's grand plan because you are too distracted by the day-to-day minutiae. You might feel as though you lack focus in your life, or you might not be able to see the higher purpose or goal of what you're doing. This can lead you to end up in meandering careers or relationships that seem to just go on without any clear trajectory or end goal. You might also experience physical symptoms. One of the most common symptoms is migraines, which affect a lot of people. You might also experience bouts of blurred vision or feelings of eye strain. When you work hard to unblock your third eye chakra, you will be able to see more clearly in order to plan your life and to connect more powerfully with your deepest intuition.

Crown Chakra

Associated Color:

White

Associated Element:

No associated element

Associated Body Parts:

The very top of the head

Description

The crown chakra is the pinnacle of all the chakras. It is the height of the chakra system and is responsible for your connection with the higher spiritual worlds. The goal of the whole chakra system is to eventually flow upward into the crown chakra, concentrating your energy there in order to achieve ultimate enlightenment. There is a lot of power to this chakra, so when or if it becomes unbalanced, it can create a lot of problems for the sufferer. You might feel constantly frustrated or cut off from your spiritual self. You might struggle with your faith or have a hard time committing to your view of the cosmic order of the universe. When this chakra is balanced, however, you will enjoy a strong connection to your higher self and gain a stronger understanding of the universe at large.

Chapter 6:
Higher Chakras

Thus far, we have only talked about the chakras that are represented on the physical body. Each chakra has a clear relationship with a particular body part and will therefore manifest in particular physical as well as psychological issues. However, there is actually another set of chakras that have an impact on how you live your life. These chakras are not located on the physical body but in spaces around the body. These are called the "higher chakras." The idea of the higher chakras is directly linked to body energy. When we talk about the body's energies, we are not just talking about actual locations on the body but the energy that your body radiates. According to the higher chakras, there are particular nodes of energy around the body that concentrate into individual chakras. This is called the "etheric body." These chakras work similarly to the rest of the body's chakras. They can become blocked or unbalanced and thus influence aspects of your thoughts and life. Again, as with the major chakras, there are a varying number of them depending on the chakra system you are using; here, we will be looking at five in particular. These five are the earth star chakra, the soul star chakra, the universal chakra, the galactic chakra, and the divine chakra. In this chapter, we will look at each of these chakras in detail and discuss their relationships with your chakra healing process.

Earth Star Chakra

Location:

Twelve inches below the feet

Description

The earth star chakra is inherently related to the root chakra. It is located below our feet and thus is almost always located within the earth. What this chakra implies is that much of our chakra energy spends time in the ground. This is a good thing! It means we have a strong connection to the earth below us and can find groundedness in its soil. So, since it's so closely related to the root chakra, what's the difference? Well, the main difference is in connection and a sense of something outside yourself, as the location of the chakra implies. This chakra focuses on your relationship with the earth below your feet, unlike the root chakra, which is more focused on your sense of identity. The earth star chakra is incredibly important not just for your sense of groundedness, but for your feelings of being a part of the organic material of the earth. It reminds us that we come from the earth and are made from its materials. We are inherently connected and will return to it one day. Your earth star chakra might also relate to your sense of mindfulness or feeling present in your day-to-day activities. Basically, the earth star chakra is your gateway to the earth below you and helps you mingle these energies together.

When your earth star chakra becomes unbalanced, you run the risk of losing this groundedness. You might feel like you are floating in space or not really human. Oftentimes, people who live lives that are very disconnected from nature experience earth star chakra blocks. For example, if you don't go for walks outside very often or if you live in an area that is very concrete-heavy, you might feel a disconnect from your earth star chakra; this can also happen if you live or work in a high-rise building and spend most of your time hundreds of feet above the earth. All of these situations are ways in which we disconnect from the earth, meaning that our earth star chakra is constantly floating around in space. To heal your earth star chakra, you should spend more time in nature to ensure that this energy node is actually making contact with the earth. Hiking, doing outdoor yoga, or even swimming in a lake can do wonders for the health of your earth star chakra.

Soul Star Chakra

Location:

Six inches above the head

Description

The soul star chakra is physically in the opposite position of your earth star chakra. It is an extension of your crown chakra just like your earth star chakra is an extension of your root chakra. The soul star chakra relates to your higher self, the core of your being that remains through reincarnations. In fact, the soul star chakra is often the path by which many people try to explore their past lives. Past lives are also known as "Akashic records" and can be used to gain powerful insight into the nature of your soul. We can carry so much from a past life that can greatly influence fears and talents in this current life. Discovering past life experiences is just as informative as discovering your childhood trauma—it can give you a lot of insight into who you are today. Some people also find that this chakra helps them to connect with their psychic side. Many people will use crystals to activate this chakra more powerfully by holding them in the spot above their heads where the soul star chakra is located. Those who have effectively opened their soul star chakra might feel as though they can see a higher plane of reality and have a stronger relationship with supernatural forces.

Universal Chakra

Location:

Twelve inches above the head

Description

Located just above the soul star chakra is the universal chakra. The universal chakra is directly related to that oneness of being we talked about in our section on Buddhism. The core energy to the universe will become available to you through the magic of the universal chakra. This chakra connects you to the unconditional love and inherent connection between all beings that pulses through the core of our world. The universal chakra also does not recognize time, so by unlocking it you can shed the oppressive shackles of linear time for something more everlasting. Crystals and crown-focused meditation can do wonders to help you unlock this chakra and start living among those cosmic realities in the great beyond.

Galactic Chakra

Location:

Two to fifteen feet above the head

Description

The galactic chakra's location surely lives up to its name being that it's the highest of the chakras we've seen so far. This chakra is further away from your body, and thus your body's energy does not have as strong an influence on it, but that does not make this chakra any less important. This chakra really allows you to connect with those intergalactic possibilities that are floating out in the universe. Some people call the galaxy chakra the "prophecy chakra." It gained such a reputation because it aids with things like divination and fortune-telling. Many professional psychics will tap into their own galactic chakras to help them connect with those future-connected forces out there in the universe. However, it is not just the future that this chakra helps with but also uncovering secret meanings and deeper truths. Psychics will also evoke their galactic chakra to help see past the debris of everyday life to the things that have not yet been revealed. If you want to have stronger insight into the future, or even achieve full-on psychic level, then you need to get actively in touch with your galactic chakra.

Divine Chakra

Location:

Above the galactic chakra to infinity

Description

The divine chakra is the highest chakra on this entire list and, in fact, the highest chakra in the entire chakra system. This chakra begins where your galactic chakra ends, assisting in your connection to important eternal forces. The divine chakra is how you connect with the highest form of knowledge and truly ascend to the uppermost point in the universe. You finally understand the oneness of everything and have completed your spiritual journey. Those who have successfully connected with their divine chakra are some of the most tranquil and zen people you will ever meet. They seem to take everything in stride as nothing seems to bother them at the roots of their being. Balance your divine chakra and you will have a life full of supreme knowledge and spiritual guidance.

Chapter 7:
Individual Chakras (Minor)

Besides the seven major chakras of the body and the five outer chakras beyond the body, there are also some less significant chakras that influence your body and behavior. These are called the "minor chakras." Some of these minor chakras are elevated to major status in certain chakra practices, but for our purposes, we will talk about them as part of the minor set. Even though they are called "minor," they can still have a significant impact on your body and mind, influencing the feelings you have or decisions you make. While the major chakras focus simply on key points in your body's core, the minor chakras are associated with more specific parts of your body. These concentrated chakra points can help you gain more specific knowledge of the body and its effect on the mind. In this chapter, we will discuss three individual minor chakras, helping you to distinguish their unique qualities and meanings. The chakras we will discuss are the foot chakra, the knee chakra, and the pubic chakra. By learning about these specific chakras, you will be able to more clearly define the areas on the body and their meanings.

The Foot Chakra

Location:

The feet

Description

The first chakra on the list of minor chakras is the foot chakra. This chakra is strongly related to the root chakra as well as the earth star chakra. In other words, it is associated with your sense of groundedness and connection to the earth. Your foot chakra is responsible for connecting your crown chakra back to the ground, thus utilizing your body as a sort of lightning rod that connects the sky energy with the ground energy. When you have a particularly blocked foot chakra, you will likely experience a lot of symptoms related to fatigue, restlessness, and disorientation. You might feel like you don't have a strong sense of home or know where your true support system lies. You might also find yourself getting frequently confused and lacking direction surrounding life plans. If you are experiencing these symptoms, then you badly need to balance your foot chakras, and the way to do this is similar to balancing the earth star chakra: Connect your feet with nature by running through grass in your bare feet or soaking them in a natural water source like a pond or spring. You can also use crystals, especially those associated with groundedness, to help unblock your foot chakras. If you are able to unblock your foot chakras and open them up to the light, then you will enjoy a life full of groundedness and certainty.

The Knee Chakra

Location:

Knees

Description

We might not think about them a lot, but our knees are actually very important parts of our body. They are the main connecting force in our legs and help us to walk properly. They are a focal point of a lot of our energy and facilitate free movement. However, like many major joints in the body, the knees also tend to be rife with problems. Many people, especially as they get older, have problems with their knees. They might have trouble walking, going up stairs, or kneeling. For this reason, it's essential to take good care of your knees and treat them well in your spiritual practice. One important way to spiritually care for your knees is through your knee chakra. This is an important minor chakra and can be used to promote energy and dynamism in your life. One of the best treatments for unblocking the knee chakra is yoga. Yoga promotes strength and connects us with the beautiful ways our bodies can move. Practicing some knee-centric yoga poses can help you to give that part of your body some love and unlock all the exciting potential at their core.

The Pubic Chakra

Location:

The genitals

Description

This chakra is a more refined version of the sacral chakra, occurring further down on the sexual organs and creating a concentrated perspective on sexuality. This chakra is solely concentrated on sexual functioning and thus touches other aspects of life such as relationships, self-esteem, and anxiety levels. Experiencing a blocked pubic chakra will inevitably lead to sexual issues, repression, or hypersexuality. This chakra can be balanced by practicing healthy attitudes toward sexuality and the body. Whether you are alone or with a partner, try to cultivate an environment in which you feel comfortable and safe. Experiment with different positions (many of which can be found in the Hindu text *Kama Sutra*) to help you with your feelings about yourself and help to unblock any frustrated sexual energy that you might be experiencing.

Pillar 3: Relationships

As we have seen throughout the previous chapters of this book, the chakras are inextricably linked to the many systems of the body as well as many other spiritual systems. Chakras do not exist in a vacuum. This is why it is so imperative that you develop a strong understanding of your chakras and the way they affect your body—because they affect many different areas of the body and mind very strongly. Now, we have already talked about chakras and their relationships to many things like religion, astrology, crystals, and other spiritual practices, but here we are going to examine two specific systems with which chakras have a very strong relationship in greater detail. In this section, we will explore this very close relationship between the chakras with one system of the body—the endocrine system—and one spiritual system—the elements. Through these comparisons, you will gain a more holistic understanding of chakras and be able to better implement them into many of the practices that you already partake in throughout your life.

Chapter 8:
Chakras and the Endocrine System

The endocrine system is interesting because it is a very important system within the body, but it doesn't get a lot of attention in the mainstream. We talk a lot about the nervous and digestive systems, which have clear functions in relation to the way we eat and manage anxiety. We are also building increasing awareness as a culture around things like the gut bacteria system and the chemical workings of mental health, but these are just a few pieces of the puzzle when we talk about all the complex systems of the body. There are so many functions the body performs without us even realizing it, and the endocrine system is one of them. Now, the endocrine system is not one hidden organ that you didn't know you had, but it is in fact a series of well-known organs that you were probably not aware had a connection to one another. This system has a very important role to play in many hormonal functions of the body. It also happens to be strongly linked with the system of the chakras and thus is relevant to bring up in a book about the subject. In this chapter, we will discuss the relationship that this system—the endocrine system—has with the chakras. First, we will give you some background on the endocrine system itself, helping you to understand its specific functions. Then, we will give you a breakdown of how this system interacts with each individual chakra as well as the chakra system as a whole.

What Is the Endocrine System?

In a way, the endocrine system is actually a kind of medicalized version of the chakras. This system divides the body up into parts, each represented on a different part of the core going from the base to the top. It also asserts that these systems are connected and, even though each performs its own specific functions, they can also greatly affect one another as well. This is what makes them a system. So, essentially, every aspect of the endocrine system has a core function, while its relationships with the other organs are expressed through the flow of hormones instead of energy. The various parts of the endocrine system thus have the same flow as chakras and are able to have as profound an impact on the mind and body. The main areas that the endocrine system deals with are metabolism, overall mental state, stress levels, pain response, energy, reproduction, and development of the body. That's a lot of aspects to preside over—important ones at that! No wonder this system is considered so important and can be seen as similar to the chakras in that way. The system consists of many organs and glands, which all have varying degrees of effects on the above list and are all required for the proper functioning of each. In short, the endocrine system is a highly important system responsible for many of the body's psychological and physiological problems.

Parts of the System

As we mentioned, there are many different organs and glands associated with the endocrine system. In many ways, this system functions similarly to that of the chakras, encompassing parts of the body from the top of the head to the bottom of the core. In this section, we will talk about the various organs of the endocrine system, detailing the way in which each one affects the body and mind as well as its relationship to the chakra system. For the sake of symmetry, we will be sorting the list from bottom to top, just like we did with the chakras, helping you to see the connections between the two systems.

Testicles/Ovaries

The first major body parts in the endocrine system are the organs that perform reproductive functions. This can be either ovaries or testicles depending on the biological sex of the person. These organs are the lowermost organs but also serve a very important function. Interestingly, these organs are not essential for survival. After all, many people have them removed or blocked off and are still perfectly healthy. However, they are necessary for some people to have in order to continue the human species. Thus, they serve an interesting function in the body—to perpetuate the human species but not the human body itself. Though they are technically the lowest organ on this list, their corresponding chakra is not actually the root chakra but the sacral chakra. This chakra presides over reproduction and, by proxy, sexual function as well. They also serve the important purpose of producing sex hormones like estrogen and testosterone in both men and women, which are hormones that help with sexual function and the development of the body. When we talk about the sacral chakra, we are thus also talking about reproduction and the ability to bring life into the world.

So, how does the dysfunction of these organs relate to the blocking of the sacral chakra? Well, the sacral chakra is also connected to creativity and self-esteem. Some people feel shame or disappointment in themselves at the inability to have children. This is something they will have to work through in order to accept themselves as they are, but nevertheless, there might be a certain bump in the road to try and recover their self-esteem. Many people also connect creativity with reproduction, viewing their children as creative projects to be sculpted properly. They might also feel the opposite way—that their creative projects are like their children. People might call their novel or film their "baby," referring to the laborious process of creation that can sometimes feel like parenting a child. Thus, reproductive dysfunction can also be metaphorically linked to creative stagnation or writer's block. In this sense, there are a lot of important physical and thematic links that connect the sacral chakra with the testicles or ovaries.

Pancreas

The pancreas is one of the more overlooked organs in the body, but it still serves a very important purpose. It is located in the abdomen just behind the stomach, and its corresponding chakra is the solar plexus. The pancreas performs one of the most important functions for the body's hormones by producing insulin, which helps to keep the body's blood sugar levels in check. It also produces hormones and helps you to digest things properly. You need your pancreas very badly. Having a dysfunctional pancreas is actually the main component of diabetes, sufferers of which are forced to regulate their blood sugar manually with synthetic insulin, which is very difficult to do and takes up a lot of time. Basically, you want your pancreas to be functioning properly.

The main way the pancreas relates to the solar plexus chakra is through its regulation of certain digestive issues. The pancreas helps to make sure your digestive system is functioning properly, which is also the main job of the solar plexus chakra. The pancreas therefore works in tandem with this chakra, meaning that blocks or malfunctions of either can have a disastrous effect on both. What you see psychologically when there are difficulties with the solar plexus chakra can also manifest in the pancreas—feelings of no control and dysregulation of the body.

This regulating organ connects strongly to the highly balance-focused solar plexus chakra.

Adrenal Gland

Another part of the endocrine system that is closely related to the solar plexus chakra is the adrenal glands. These are glands that sit on top of both of your kidneys and help them to perform their main functions. These glands are also strongly connected to other glands within the body's system, such as the pituitary gland and the hypothalamus. These three glands form their own mini-endocrine system, helping the body to regulate many different essential hormones. In particular, the adrenal gland is responsible for distributing hormones such as epinephrine, which is also known as adrenaline. Adrenaline is responsible for your body's energy levels and can give you that important energy boost and sense of vigor in times of extreme stress. What these hormonal functions essentially accomplish is the regulation of things like blood pressure and metabolism. These are two highly essential aspects of the body, the mismanagement of which can result in some serious chronic issues that can eventually lead to fatal problems like heart disease. We can see how both of the organs that we have talked about so far in relation to the solar plexus chakra are highly connected to regulation. These organs help the body maintain balance, which is again strongly related to the solar plexus's functions.

Thymus

Moving up on the body, the thymus is located in the chest. I'm sure you can already surmise which chakra is connected with this organ: the heart chakra. The thymus performs some very important functions in the body's immune system. When you are fighting a virus, your thymus is the one fighting against the body's invaders. It helps keep you healthy and strong. This is related to the heart chakra's focus on health and happiness, especially around family. You can think of your body as a family and your thymus as the protective parent trying to keep danger away. It's an organ of nurturing and is essential in helping you stay strong against many different illnesses that can potentially attack the body and cause great harm.

Thyroid

The thyroid is located just by the voice box at the front of the neck. Because of its location, it is of course directly related to the throat chakra. The thyroid is responsible for your metabolism. Many people with thyroid dysfunctions have a lot of trouble maintaining a healthy weight, often remaining underweight despite a healthy diet or overweight despite calorie restrictions. Many people with thyroid issues, particularly those that are undiagnosed, feel that they are out of control of their bodies and might experience self-esteem issues as a result. A dysregulated thyroid can also lead to chronic anxiety issues, so many people with thyroid issues might experience social withdrawal or extreme anxiety around things like speaking in public. Interestingly, this has many parallels to some of the issues outlined in our section on an unbalanced throat chakra. If you find that you are experiencing extreme anxiety, then you might have a problem with either your throat chakra or your thyroid.

Hypothalamus

Finally, we reach the brain and thus the third eye chakra. The hypothalamus is a gland within the brain that is responsible for a wide variety of brain functions. It is located directly below the optic nerve, which physically links it very closely with the third eye chakra's relationship to sight. There are many things it does though—much more than anything related to sight. The hypothalamus controls things like your blood pressure, appetite, general body temperature regulation, and even sleep. All of these things are very important. Most significantly, all of these regulations feed back into your cognitive function. Things like having high blood pressure, an unregulated eating schedule, or not getting enough sleep all have a significant negative impact on the brain and its function, but of course, if the brain is not functioning properly, then these things aren't either. We can see the vicious cycle the hypothalamus can get into if it is not regulated. This also connects to the long-term goals and planning of the third eye chakra. Regulating these foundational functions of the body helps to keep your body healthy and your mind sharp and has a strong effect on the way you think.

Breakdown of the Chakra Connection

The connection between the chakra points and the key organs of the endocrine system is certainly striking. It seems that even before we had the technology to dissect the human body, we were acutely aware of the fact that these points were very important to an interconnected web. By comparing the endocrine system to the chakra system, we can see that the system of the chakras actually has a sound medical basis. These points on the body are not chosen at random, and we can see how they actually have similar functions to the body's overall purpose. We can also see how the chakras have a strong connection to the actual functions of the body, and we can observe the specific ways in which a blocked chakra can affect the body. This is not to say that chakra healing needs medical science to legitimize it but merely to point out that they do not come from nowhere and their relationship to the body can be observed as well as felt.

Chapter 9:
Chakras and the Elements

Back in our section on individual chakras, we listed an element that coincides with each chakra. This might not have seemed that important at the time, but the connection with the elements is one of the things that links the chakras to many other spiritual systems. The elements each carry meanings associated with them that can help further inform your chakra healing practice. Additionally, linking the elements in your chakras to the elemental associations of other spiritual practices such as astrology, crystal healing, and tarot can help you incorporate these other practices into your chakra healing. In this chapter, we will talk about the association between the elements and the chakras. First, we will give a detailed definition of the specific elemental system we will be using so you understand the specifics of this system and where it came from. Next, we will list each individual element and give you a description of all the things it is associated with as well as the specific sides of each spiritual practice it presides over.

What Are the Elements?

First of all, let's identify what elements we are talking about here. You might be familiar with the periodic table of elements, which you may have learned about in chemistry class. This system is an ever-expanding chart of every single chemical that human beings have discovered on Earth so far. However, we will not be discussing this system of elements. Instead, we will be focusing on ancient elemental systems that were developed before things like microscopes could reveal more division among the elements. One such elemental system, which is probably the most famous of the ancient ones, is the Greek system of the four elements. These elements are earth, fire, water, and air. They feature very prominently throughout ancient Greek science, philosophy, and astrology. Systems like the zodiac, tarot cards, and crystal healing are all designed to correspond to one of these four elements. For this reason, you can often divide many of these spiritual systems into groups of four to help you distinguish or specialize your healing practice. However, again, this is not quite the system we will be talking about. In chakra healing, there are actually five elements. The first four are earth, fire, water, and air, similar to the Greek system, but the Hindu or chakra element system includes a fifth element called "ether," or space. This element has a higher connection and does not necessarily map onto other spiritual systems in the same way, though it does map onto the chakras. Each chakra relates to one of these elements, except the top two which don't have elemental connections. In the rest of this chapter, we will look at the five elements of the chakras, explaining both their meanings and their connections.

Earth

Ah, the Earth. Our home, our protector. Feeding us, sheltering us, clothing us. It's no wonder people nickname the Earth "mother." In a way, the Earth gave birth to us all. Though most of the elements on the periodic table are found in the earth, in this system it is a whole element in itself. In most spiritual systems, the earth is associated with a grounding force. You can think of the earth as either things that are associated with the ground, such as plants, dirt, or rocks, or you can think of this element as the core of the Earth itself. Whichever is easier for you to visualize is best. Most people feel a strong connection to the earth, especially if you are someone who has powerful feelings of connectedness or belonging. Thus, in most spiritual systems, the earth is in some way associated with rootedness or down-to-earth qualities. In the chakra system, the earth is associated with the root chakra, as we talked about back in Chapter 5. Here, we will look at all the spiritual systems that include the earth and explore how it interacts with your chakra healing journey.

Associated Zodiac Signs

Virgo, Taurus, and Capricorn are the signs on the zodiac that are associated with the earth. These are all signs that are known for being very practical and straightforward. There is no messing with earth signs since they tend to see through to the truth of everything. If you have earth in your sun sign or birth month, then you will probably be a highly pragmatic person, very protective of your loved ones, and might even feel a particular connection to earthly things in general. If you are experiencing a root chakra block, look at some of the earth signs that might be in your birth chart. Your sun, moon, or some of your planets might be in earth signs, which can help you gain insight into your connection to your root chakra and this element in general. You also might want to coordinate your chakra healing practices around earth signs in the sky. Consider waiting until an earth sign birth month to start your chakra healing journey. Making this connection with your chakras and your birth chart, as well as the current celestial sky, can help you specify and clarify your chakra healing practice.

Associated Crystals

Many crystals involved in healing have significant associations with the earth. This makes sense as most crystals are mined out of the ground and therefore come from the earth. Three of the main earth-associated crystals are tiger's eye, smoky quartz and amazonite. Tiger's eye is particularly useful for giving you energy and confidence. If you feel insecure in your grounding energy, a tiger's eye can help you reconnect with your self-esteem. Smoky quartz, on the other hand, is a protective stone, both against actual illness and negative energy in general. This crystal is perfect if you want to build a deeper connection with the earth. Finally, amazonite is strongly associated with material abundance. This might not seem like it is associated with the earth, but as we will see below in the tarot section, abundance is actually related to crop success, which is connected to the earth. Using crystals associated with the earth can really help you with unblocking or opening up your root chakra. If you have a root chakra block, consider using one of these three crystals in your meditation practice to give it some attention.

Associated Tarot Suit

Tarot is another popular spiritual practice. Tarot cards are similar to conventional playing cards in the sense that there are four suits, each of which has a set of number and face cards. The suits, however, are different in a tarot deck. Instead of diamonds, hearts, clubs, and spades, you have pentacles, cups, wands, and swords. People use these cards to gain insight into their lives and futures. The four suits are also associated with specific elements. The other major difference between tarot cards and other card decks is that there are two parts to the deck: the major arcana and the minor arcana. The minor arcana is the four suits with their number and face cards—the part of the deck that most resembles a conventional deck—totaling 56 cards. The major arcana is a series of individual cards which don't belong to a particular suit but relate to archetypes or ideas. You might have even seen some cards in popular culture, such as death, the hermit, or the hanged man. Some of these cards have elemental associations, so we will include those in our chakra discussion as well as the suit cards.

In this case, the suit in a tarot deck that is most associated with the earth is pentacles. Pentacles are gold coins that symbolize money and prosperity in the world. As we said above, money and material prosperity have long been associated with the earth, dating back to the days of widespread agriculture. People's money quite literally came out of the ground and so the association was born. For this reason, many tarot decks feature nature-based themes and colors in the artwork for their pentacle suit. There are several ways to incorporate tarot practice into your chakra healing. You can inquire as to whether there might be a root chakra block in the first place by doing a reading for yourself or going to a professional psychic and taking notice if a lot of pentacles are coming up in your reading, especially if they are reversed, as this may indicate a blockage. If you already feel like you are experiencing a blockage, you can try an isolated reading. Some tarot readers will isolate parts of the deck, such as a single suit, to try and determine a particular problem. You could try an isolated reading with just the pentacles to get a more specific idea of your relationship to the earth element. You can also see if any earth-associated major arcana cards come up. Some major arcana cards that are connected with the earth element include the devil, the hierophant, the empress, the hermit, and the world. Using these methods, you can employ the tarot to help you both ascertain and improve your relationship with the earth.

Water

The next element we will be talking about is water. Water is the element most closely associated with flow as is represented by the fluid currents of the ocean or the meandering trajectory of a brook. We are just as connected to the element of water as we are to that of earth. First of all, our bodies are about 70% water, meaning that water makes up the vast majority of what is inside us. Furthermore, we need to drink water in order to survive, cook food, bathe ourselves, wash things for protection from disease, and even navigate the world. Water has a huge impact on not only individual human lives but on entire civilizations. Most major cities in the world were built on a coast or a river, ensuring that every inhabitant had an adequate water source. This element is thus extremely important to us. The chakra most linked to water is the next one up from the root chakra—the sacral chakra. This chakra is tied to water through its focus on inner emotions and sexuality. In this section, we will look at how water figures into other spiritual systems as well as its impact on the sacral chakra.

Associated Zodiac Signs

Similar to how there are three earth signs in the 12-sign zodiac system, there are also three water signs. These water signs are Pisces, Cancer, and Scorpio. All three of these signs are known for being very emotional. Pisces are emotional in a sensitive way, being extremely self-conscious and vulnerable to criticism. Cancers, on the other hand, are more emotional in the way that they are very focused on love and family and protective of those they love. Finally, Scorpios are emotional but in a very secretive way. They hold their cards close to their chests and take a long time to let people in. We can see this play out in the sacral chakra, especially with some of the extremely intimate relationships the sacral chakra covers. This chakra is associated with some of the most sensitive and vulnerable emotions, especially when they are related to sexuality and the most inner self. As we said in the above section on earth, you can use the water-associated zodiac signs to help time your sacral chakra healing practice by either locating them on your birth chart or performing your healing practice at times when that sign is in sun or moon.

Associated Crystals

Most of the crystals associated with the element of water are focused on bringing you inner peace and fostering healthy relationships with the people in your life. Three of the main water-associated crystals are aquamarine, turquoise, and amethyst. Aquamarine is a calming crystal. This crystal is designed to create a sense of tranquility within your life and, by proxy, help reduce stress and anxiety. It is also helpful for focusing your energies. Turquoise, on the other hand, is a powerful cleansing stone. This crystal is especially useful for banishing negative energy from your life which, in the context of relationships, might mean cutting out some particularly toxic people. Finally, amethyst is a healing stone particularly useful for emotional trauma. It can help soothe those wounds that you might have endured throughout your life and help you to rebuild a new life. If you are suffering from a block in your sacral chakra, then you can use one of these three crystals in your healing practice to help open it up.

Associated Tarot Suit

The tarot suit associated with water is cups. The cups of the suit are designed to hold water, and whether or not they are full, or the degree to which they are full, is often laden with meaning within the deck. Often, illustrations for the cups suit will feature water in other places as well, not just inside the cups. Some of the most common motifs are a waterfall or river. These symbolize new beginnings but also an abundance of love or emotional energy. The major arcana cards that are associated with water include the moon, the priestess, the chariot, the hanged man, and death. With your sacral chakra, you want to be able to open yourself up to the most intimate parts of this energy. Do a tarot reading, either with the whole deck or just the cups, and see what comes up. If you are getting a lot of reversed water cards or negative water cards, such as the five of cups, then you might have an imbalanced sacral chakra. Use the readings to construct a path toward opening that chakra.

Fire

The third element on this list is fire. As you can probably guess, fire is often strongly associated with passion, confidence, and boldness. It can also be associated with creativity, being the spark or the light bulb that enlightens the creative mind. And of course, it is also associated with sexuality, especially when people speak of the fires of passion or a burning desire. This element is, perhaps unexpectedly, associated with the solar plexus chakra. This chakra connects with the driven aspect of fire which forms a large part of your self-esteem. Fire also connects to some of the physical properties of the solar plexus chakra, which some refer to as your "digestive fire." In this section, we will look at how the element of fire relates to your solar plexus chakra and its themes in other spiritual practices.

Associated Zodiac Signs

Fire is very important to some of the zodiac signs. The signs that are under the influence of fire are Leo, Aries, and Sagittarius. Leo is the sign of confidence and social influence. Basically, Leos just can't help but be charming. This relates to the social connection aspect of the solar plexus chakra. Aries is the sign of competition. Aries love to spar with people in a friendly (or not-so-friendly!) manner, which connects to the desire to perform well that sits at the core of the solar plexus chakra. And Sagittarians are known for their ability to mediate, which can provide a different perspective on the social personalities of Leo and Aries. Therefore, we can see that these fire-associated signs in the zodiac have a lot in common with the solar plexus chakra and can thus be used in tandem with your chakra healing process. Timing your solar plexus chakra healing with one of these three signs will help you align with the fire element more closely and create a more focused healing practice.

Associated Crystals

Crystal healing can help you greatly with balancing your solar plexus chakra, especially ones that have a strong association with fire. Three of the best crystals to use in your solar plexus chakra healing journey are garnet, red jasper, and carnelian. Garnet is one of the most potent and powerful crystals. It is strongly associated with love and relationships as well as balancing your sexual self. It is also associated with perseverance and forward momentum, which resonates with the social achievement aspect of the solar plexus chakra. Red jasper is more of a calming, protective crystal. This gemstone has the ability to balance your intense emotions and bring a sense of tranquility to your life. It is also a great manifestation crystal, helping you to bring positive energy into your life. Finally, carnelian is one of the best success-bringing crystals, resonating with the confidence and drive you are trying to manifest through your solar plexus chakra. Using any of these three crystals in your meditation or chakra practice will help you link better with the fire element and your solar plexus chakra more specifically.

Associated Tarot Suit

The suit in the tarot most associated with fire is wands. This might be a strange association, but the wand is meant to represent spark and creativity, with magical fire pouring out of its tip. Usually, the wand suit is used to talk about your feelings toward creativity or even professional pursuits. We can see this reflected in the way the solar plexus chakra is often linked to our social pursuits and self-esteem in relation to how we are perceived by others. Some of the major arcana cards associated with the element of fire are the sun, the tower, the emperor, and the wheel of fortune. If you want to learn more about your relationship with your solar plexus chakra, then you can do some tarot readings and focus on the placement of the wand suit and the above-mentioned major arcana cards in your reading.

Air

Coming to the final of the Greek elements, we have air. Air is, of course, the lightest element, consisting mainly of gas. As with the other elements, air is also necessary to sustain life. Air not only nourishes us by giving us oxygen to breathe in and power our bodies with, but it sustains many other things as well, like plants and animals. It's no coincidence, then, that the chakra most associated with air is the one right next to our lungs: the heart chakra. Physically, the oxygen we breathe from air is one of the most important aspects of powering our physical hearts, so air as an element is quite literally involved with this part of our bodies. Moreover, air is also metaphorically linked to our heart chakras, representing the expansiveness and higher knowledge of unconditional love. In this section, we will look at the ways in which the element of air intersects with aspects of other spiritual systems and how to harness it in order to help you on your chakra journey.

Associated Zodiac Signs

The three zodiac signs associated with the element of air are Gemini, Libra, and Aquarius. These three signs all have strong associations with malleability as a person. This might seem like a bad thing since we tend to think of people who hold steadfast to their beliefs as stronger; however, this malleability can also be a strength, allowing these air signs to make compromises and be more open-minded in order to help those they love and adopt new worldviews. When healing your heart chakra, look at the qualities of the air signs and connect with some of the ones in your birth chart or that are in the current sky's chart.

Associated Crystals

Despite being rocks from the ground, there are actually many crystals that have a strong association with the air. Three of the best crystals to use for air-connected heart chakra healing are fluorite, clear quartz, and blue lace agate. Fluorite is a great crystal for promoting more focused, rational thinking. In the context of the heart chakra, this can help you bring clarity to your relationships and perhaps help you evaluate which ones are important. Clear quartz is also useful for clarity, but it is also considered to be the leader of the crystals, so to speak. You can use this crystal in tandem with other crystals to create a lightness and clarity in your manifestation of chakra healing practice. Blue lace agate is a tranquilizing stone that helps you to bring a sense of peace to your life. All these crystals are excellent for strengthening your connection to the air element and your heart chakra.

Associated Tarot Suit

The tarot suit associated with the element of air is swords. Swords are the suit of enlightenment and sharp rational thinking. Often, illustrations on cards in the sword suit will feature clouds, birds, or the sky very prominently. Many tarot readers will interpret this suit as being related to both your academic pursuits, if that is relevant, as well as your higher thoughts or spiritual pursuits. This is the suit in which you will find clarity of mind and where logic will prevail. The major arcana cards associated with the element of air are the fool, the lovers, the magician, and the star. When you are using this suit in relation to your heart chakra, you can evaluate the place of these logical ideas and higher realities within your relationships as well as at the core of your being.

Ether

Now that we have completed the four Greek elements, we can move on to the three additional Vedic, or Hindu, elements. These higher elements are different from the previous four in the sense that they do not have a physical reality. They also do not feature prominently outside of Vedic philosophy, which is why they don't have corresponding tarot cards, crystals, or zodiac signs. From here on out, we will simply describe the element as it pertains to the relevant chakra and what it means for connecting with that chakra or opening it up.

The first of the higher three elements we will be looking at is ether, or empty space. This is essentially the absence of physical matter. It's what you would get if you sucked out all the air from the space around us. This element is actually very important to Vedic philosophy since it is thought to be the first element ever created. It is the empty space into which the universe expanded and thus is the base for all life. However, this element does not just exist in empty spaces but in fact all around us; thus, it is the linking force between all things in the universe. The connecting chakra to the element of ether is the throat chakra. The way that this chakra connects to ether is through the theme of authenticity. Because of the extreme clarity of emptiness, there is no room for bamboozlement. Channeling this element can help you if you have blocks with your throat chakra, clearing the air for you to live a more honest and authentic life.

Light

Recently, quantum physics has been doing a lot of research into the behavior of light in physical space. Light travels through things called photons, but physicists still can't agree on whether photons are particles or waves. This ambiguity is what makes photons so interesting. Photons are also extremely fast. In fact, the speed of light is the highest recorded speed in the universe. This element is thus perfect for association with the third eye chakra. The third eye chakra is all about enlightenment, stretching the boundaries of everyday perception. Light is the element that makes sight possible. Everything you see is actually just different colors and shades of light, and thus your eyes work merely as light receptors. Metaphorical light, or enlightenment, also forms a connection between the third eye chakra and the element of light. Consider connecting with different light sources in your life to help unblock your third eye chakra. Evaluate how much natural versus artificial light you use in your daily life and perhaps try to use more natural light. You could even try to change up your light sources by introducing a new light source. Try meditating by moonlight to recalibrate your body and your third eye chakra's relationship with light.

Thought

The final and most immaterial element on this list is thought. Although scientists mainly talk about thought as a series of neurological connections, almost every spiritual philosophy categorizes the human mind or soul as being separate from the physical body. Thus, thought in this context is immaterial thought—not the workings of neurons. This element cannot be measured, seen, or even perceived by anyone other than the thinker, and this is why it is ultimately strongly connected to the crown chakra, which is all about the highest realities of our minds and our connection to the universe beyond. This is why mindfulness is such an important aspect of enlightenment and spiritual healing. It allows us to truly focus and be at one with our thoughts, allowing them to pass by us and be noticed without being sources of stress. If you want to learn to balance your crown chakra, you need to put a strong emphasis on your thoughts and the ways in which they connect with the outside world and the universe at large.

The 6 Pillars of Chakra Healing

Pillar 4: Activation

Now that you understand all about chakras, their history, their individual meanings, and the connections they have to your physical body and other spiritual systems, you are ready to start learning about the actual process of using them to heal. This is the point in the book where we move away from theory toward a more practical approach to the chakras. In this pillar, we will talk about all the different ways you can start to activate your chakras. In the first chapter of the pillar, we will talk about the benefits of opening and activating your chakras. This section will list the reasons why you should care for your chakras, all the hidden problems that can arise when they are blocked, and what opening them up can do for your life. In the second chapter of this pillar, we will talk about the specific ways you can activate your chakras, helping you begin your journey of chakra healing. Throughout this section, we will make a strong case for why and how you can start activating your chakras for a more fulfilled life.

Chapter 10:
Why Should You Open Your Chakras?

Throughout this book, you have probably been wondering about the specific reasons you should be balancing your chakras. After all, you've gone your whole life without even knowing about them, so what's the big deal? Well, as you might have ascertained throughout the last few chapters, there are actually a lot of compelling reasons as to why you should be trying to activate, or open, your chakras. Your chakras are gateways to your body and mind, useful tools for understanding and remedying many of the difficulties you might be facing throughout your life. In this chapter, we will be outlining some of the most compelling ways in which chakras can help enhance your life. First, we will discuss how chakras can help you pinpoint issues in your life that you might previously have struggled to recognize and articulate. Next, we will look at how chakras can greatly enhance your relationship with yourself and your sense of personhood. After that, we will talk about how you can enhance your general spiritual life by incorporating chakra practice. And finally, we will discuss how chakras forge a strong mind-body connection that will help you bring these forces together. By the end of this chapter, you'll be ready to start activating your chakras!

Target Issues in Your Life

Many people experience problems in their lives that they may not be able to really explain or put their finger on. It could be a mysterious physical problem that doesn't have a clear cause, such as migraines or chronic fatigue, or it could be a psychological problem like depression or anxiety. For these vaguer conditions, many people go through the medical system without getting a definitive answer about their condition from doctors; thus, many people end up very frustrated by their conditions and begin looking elsewhere for answers. What chakra healing does is break down the body into parts and help you identify where on the body your ailment might be originating. For example, if you have persistent headaches, it might relate to your third eye chakra being imbalanced, or if you have a lot of anxiety around speaking in public or meeting new people, it could be caused by a block in your throat chakra. The ability to pinpoint the exact causes or location of your issue can be a dream come true for sufferers of vague or unidentified illnesses. Chakra healing can help people with this very thing because it creates a clear system of division in their body, helping to identify and connect more specific problems.

Learn About Yourself

Connecting with your chakras can also teach you a lot about yourself. If you have certain personality traits that are linked to a particular chakra, then you might be able to investigate why that particular chakra is important. Notice if any of the other qualities of that chakra resonate with you so that you can see the impact it might have had on you and your life. By investigating aspects of the chakras, you might also have noticed that there were certain chakras you connected with more than others and possibly some things that may have triggered particular anxieties. In this case, you will be able to see what areas of your life might need more work and attention. The chakras help you with this because they compartmentalize different aspects of life, perhaps pointing out areas that we might not have thought of. To aid in this aspect of chakra healing, consider going through each chakra one at a time and really evaluating your relationship to that area of your life as well as any physical symptoms you tend to experience related to the particular chakra.

Enhance Other Spiritual Practices

As we talked about back in Chapter 9, there are many other spiritual practices that have elemental links to the chakras. However, the connections go far beyond merely associating with similar elements. Almost every other spiritual practice in existence can be enhanced through the amalgamation of chakras. Things like mindfulness, meditation, tarot readings, and astrological practice can all benefit from a thorough knowledge of your chakras. Mindfulness can help chakras by focusing on specific areas of the body in your meditative practice. Likewise, meditation also benefits from a more focused approach and especially an awareness of the higher chakras that are meant to connect you with the universe at large. Having a keen awareness and openness toward your upper chakras will vastly improve your meditative experience and help you reach higher spiritual enlightenment through it. Tarot and astrology might also become more clear once your chakras are activated, helping you to see how different aspects of your birth chart relate to your chakras or how tarot readings might interact with them, helping you to make better decisions for the future. Crystals, too, can benefit from activated chakras. The more awake your chakras are, the more receptive your body is to crystal energy, and thus the more effective your crystal healing practice will become. Whatever combination of practices you are engaging in, you will certainly benefit from activated chakras.

Strengthen Mind-Body Connection

Finally, chakras are all about the inherent connections between the body and the mind. Your understanding and concept of your body will fundamentally change after the inclusion of chakra healing into your practice. Most of us walk around with a sort of harsh mind-body division. We think of our body as simply a machine performing the baser functions and our brain as the thing that has the most profound impact on our lives, where all the important stuff happens. But through chakra healing, you can really see how both physiological and psychological processes are stored in the brain and the body. You can then develop a stronger connection between these two. Activating your chakras will help you create a reciprocal healing process in which you can heal your mind through your body and your body through your mind. Perhaps targeting your physical stomach with a healthier diet can actually help your social anxiety. Conversely, working on your social anxiety with a therapist might help cure your chronic stomachaches. Chakra healing gives you the tools to make these connections and allows you to work toward a more holistic healing practice for yourself. By activating your specific chakras, you are awakening this connection, meaning that your old dichotomy between the intellectual workings of your mind and the basic functions of the body will be no more. You can enjoy a strong connection as well as more opportunities for growth!

Chapter 11:
How to Awaken Your Chakras

Okay, you're convinced—activating your chakras is important! But how do you actually do it? What are the processes whereby you can start to actually awaken your chakras? Likely, this is the moment you've been waiting for as you've been reading this book. Though we have discussed some chakra-opening methods already, such as using crystals or astrology, we have not yet discussed the actual process behind the opening of the chakras themselves in isolation. Well, in this chapter, we will be discussing exactly how you can activate your chakras. First, we will explore what actually happens when your chakras become activated to help you be able to judge the difference between an activated and unactivated chakra. Then, we will look at a step-by-step approach to opening up your chakras. We will guide you through the actual stages, starting with the root chakra and ending with the crown chakra. Though we will not be touching on the other sets of chakras we mentioned earlier in this book, many of the ideas we will be talking about will help you in case you do want to move on to activating those other chakras. By the end of this chapter, you should be all ready to start using some techniques for opening your chakras!

What Happens When Chakras Are Activated?

First of all, what does an opened chakra feel like? Because the chakras allow you to look at a specific aspect of your body and life, you will have a better idea of how they feel because you can laser focus on just that one area. There are two aspects to the feeling of a chakra being either opened or closed: the body and the mind. In the body, you will likely feel less tension in that area if the chakra is open. You might be relieved of bad neck muscle tension, for instance, after balancing your throat chakra, or you might have relief from constipation after balancing your root chakra. You might also feel a stronger connection to that body part and be relieved of shame about it. The second aspect is the mind, which connects to the facet of life over which the individual chakra presides. If you are able to unblock your chakra in that area, that part of your life should see some improvement. You might notice a more active appetite for healthier foods by balancing your solar plexus chakra or a greater capacity for care by balancing your heart chakra. Ensuring that you know very well how to balance these areas of your life will help you to see growth and change. When you successfully open all your chakras, you will be able to facilitate the energy flow between your root and crown chakras. This creates a sense of fluidity and helps your chakras work together toward a more holistic approach to health and happiness.

Where Do You Start?

All this advice might seem overwhelming, especially if you are not sure which chakras you need to be balancing. You have likely already done some reflection about this, but even so, it's hard to know for sure as there is some crossover of symptoms, especially psychological symptoms. For example, struggles with self-esteem can manifest through the root, sacral, or even solar plexus chakras. Therefore, even if you have strong insight into your individual issues, you still might not be completely clear as to the chakras that need activation. From there, you have two options. You can either isolate one or a few chakras that you think need work and follow the process of activating just those. This is advisable for those who already have a good idea of what their chakra needs look like, having narrowed it down to just one or two individual chakras as the source of their issues. Alternatively, you can do a full-body chakra heal. This is where you start from your root chakra and focus on each chakra in sequence until you reach your crown chakra. This is advisable to do if you're not sure what the sources of your chakra difficulties are or if you want a more holistic healing process. It's also advisable that you do this every so often. After all, just because you aren't having an issue with a particular chakra doesn't mean it couldn't use some attention. Therefore, you should do a full-body chakra heal if you haven't identified the source of your chakra issues as well as periodically to promote the health of all your chakras and to support the connections between them. In the next section, we will go chakra by chakra, giving you the best ways to balance those individual areas for a better quality of life.

Chakra by Chakra

Because each of your chakras is responsible for a different area of your body and life, they all need to be approached in a slightly different way. In this section, we will look at the different methods you can use to help heal your chakras and make sure they are taken care of properly. These methods will all involve simply your body and your mind, so no materials are necessary! However, if you want to use some aids, they certainly can help enhance your chakra healing process. There are two main types of aids people use for their chakra sessions. The first kind is environmental aids. These are simply things you can do to your room to put yourself in a relaxed, contemplative, or meditative mood. This can be anything that helps you relax, such as candles, soft lighting, or instrumental atmospheric music. These things are not essential but can certainly make the process better than trying to do chakra awakenings in a crowded room or brightly lit space! Basically, this kind of aid is about finding your comfort zone so you can do the difficult work of activating your chakras without distractions or added stress. The other kind of aid is spiritual aids, such as the ones we talked about in Chapter 9. If you are into another spiritual practice, such as crystals, incorporating that practice into your chakra healing can actually do a lot for your connection to your chakras. Since you already have a strong connection to your crystals, for instance, you can have an even stronger connection to your chakras by combining the practices. This aspect isn't necessary either, but it can enhance the experience if that sort of thing is important to you. In this section, however, we will just give you aid-less techniques to which you can add these aids if you wish. We will go from the root to the crown to help you envision the process as a cohesive sequence.

Root

To activate the root chakra, you can engage in some simple meditation. This isn't just any meditation, however, it is the kind of prototypical meditation you will often see in advertisements for yoga classes. This posture involves sitting cross-legged on the ground and putting your hands on your knees in the "okay" position facing up, your thumb and index finger pointing toward the sky. This hand position is called a "mudra" and is very important in Hindu philosophy. Sitting cross-legged on the ground is essential for accessing your root chakra as it creates a connection between your body, specifically the root chakra, and the earth. Some modifications can be to sit cross-legged with your nondominant leg on top, just to build better awareness in your body, or to sit in the lotus position or upside-down crossed legs to build some stretching into the process. For the best results, you should do this outside, actually touching the earth, but if that is not an option, pick the lowest floor in your home that you have access to so you are as close to the earth as possible. Another aspect of this posture is the chant. You should build a chant into your root chakra healing process. One of the ideal ones is "lam," which you can chant over and over. Try to really lose yourself in the chant and feel the vibrations of your voice in your root chakra. Doing this exercise regularly can help you to build a stronger connection to your root chakra and hopefully work on activating the best of its powers.

Sacral

This chakra, which is located slightly above your root chakra, should be activated with a slightly different pose. This pose involves sitting on your knees with your heels underneath you. Place your hands on your knees, palms up. This is another mudra that is connected to the sacral chakra. Try to focus your mind on your sacral chakra area as well as any concerns you have that you know are directly related to the health of your sacral chakra. The chant that goes along with the sacral chakra position is "vam," which you should chant while you are in this pose. Just as with your root chakra exercise, this should help to stimulate your sacral chakra and hopefully build a stronger connection between your mind, your body, and the spiritual energy of that chakra.

Solar Plexus

To activate your solar plexus chakra, you should assume the same pose that you did with your sacral chakra—sitting on your knees. However, this time your hand position will be different. Instead of on your knees, you should rest your hands on your stomach, directly touching your solar plexus chakra. You should also incorporate the specific chant that goes along with the solar plexus chakra, which is "ram." Again, try to lose yourself in this chant and feel its vibrations in your solar plexus chakra. Connecting these areas of your body should help stimulate energy flow into the solar plexus chakra and remove some of the blockages that might have arisen within them.

Heart

The next position on this list involves sitting on a chair. Because this chakra is higher on the body, you want to physically raise yourself off the floor to symbolize its higher energy. However, because it is also in the middle of the body and not the top, you are not standing all the way up but instead creating a halfway point. This aspect of the heart chakra posture ensures that you will be channeling the intermediary energy of the heart chakra. Besides sitting on a chair, there is also a mudra associated with this chakra. It involves both hands: Simply place your thumbs together and your index fingers together to form a sort of diamond in front of your chest. Assume this mudra while you are sitting to help channel the energy of the heart chakra. You should also incorporate your chant. In this case, the chant is the word "yam." Hold this posture and try to feel the energy flowing through your heart chakra.

Throat

To activate your throat chakra, you are going to go back to the same position you were in for the sacral and solar plexus chakras. This time, though, there is no corresponding mudra. Instead, you are to focus on elongating your body, especially your neck. Straighten your back and look slightly up and ahead. This helps open up the physical space of your neck, leaving room for spiritual energy to flow throughout. You should also close your eyes to help facilitate your concentration in this pose. The chant associated with the throat chakra is "ham," which you should try to feel especially clearly in your voice box. After all, this chakra is especially about speech, so your chant will be particularly important. Try to feel all that negative verbal energy spilling out, making way for more positive communication.

Third Eye

The pose you want to assume for your third eye chakra is a cross between those for the root and throat chakras. You want to sit down cross-legged, with your back elongated and your eyes closed. This time, closing your eyes is especially spiritually connected to making way for other forms of knowledge to enter your head and to practice seeing with your mind rather than just your blunt senses. The chant for the third eye chakra is simply "om," a chant you have likely already heard of in connection to conventional meditation. Activating your third eye chakra can be achieved using this pose.

Crown

Finally, for your crown chakra, you want to assume a posture similar to the previous one but this time sitting cross-legged on a chair. This gives you the same raised quality as with the position for the heart chakra, but it still incorporates postures from the other chakras, signifying the unity within the chakra system. The final chant for the crown chakra is the same as for the third eye, "om," again borrowing from the previous chakras to symbolize the crown chakra as being above all the others. Using all or some of these poses can be an amazing way to truly activate your chakras and lead you toward a more dynamic relationship with their power.

Pillar 5: Balance

Besides activating your chakras, there are other aspects of them that need to be accounted for. As we have reiterated throughout this book, your chakras are meant to work together as a system. They have unique qualities individually, but they don't exist in isolation from one another. First of all, the energy flow that we've been talking about makes it so that all of your chakras need to be activated and opened in order to work at their fullest potential individually. However, it is also necessary for your chakras to be in balance with one another, to share common vibrations. You can think of this as similar to a home entertainment system. Even if you have the best devices—speakers, screen, Blu-ray player, and so on—they still need to all be connected to the same Wi-Fi and hooked up to one another in order to create that cohesive system. It's the same with chakras. Not only do they all need to be activated, but they also all need to be in line with one another in order for the entire unit to work as it should. In this pillar, we will shift into a discussion of the chakras as a balancing act. First, we will look into how to evaluate the relative balancing of your chakras, examining how you can tell whether your chakras are blocked or unbalanced. In the next chapter, we will instruct you on how to actually go through the process of balancing your chakras. By the end of this pillar, you should clearly understand the distinct qualities of chakra balancing and know how to do it properly.

Chapter 12:
What Is Chakra Balancing?

Alright, so now you know that chakra balancing is different from chakra activating, but what exactly is it? Well, the main idea of chakra balancing is that it is possible for chakras to be overactive as well as underactive. While it might seem positive for your chakras to be overactive, meaning they are working harder, it isn't necessarily a good thing. In fact, a chakra being overactive is often a sign that your chakras are overall unbalanced. Sometimes when a chakra is underactive, it means that other chakras are leaned on harder. You can think of the chakras as classmates working together on a group project. When everyone is putting in equal effort, then no one should be doing more than their share since the slack is being picked up equally. However, if there are those who are underperforming, skipping group meetings, or not completing their portions of the task, then often the other people will have to overperform, doing more than their due because they need to overcompensate for their classmate's failings. You can see this kind of dynamic played out more subtly within people themselves. Sometimes, when a person feels like they are underperforming at something, they will try to overcompensate in other areas. So, kids who struggle in school might try extra hard at sports, or kids who don't fit in might cultivate an artistic persona outside of school to gain self-esteem. In this sense, we can see how chakras being blocked or underperforming might cause other chakras to become overactive in compensation. You can boost those underperforming or blocked chakras by activating them, but often you will also need to learn not to rely on your other chakras so much to stop them from having to overperform and ensure that your chakras are all functioning equally and in tandem with one another.

What Is the Difference Between Balancing and Activating?

In the previous pillar, we only discussed chakras as being either blocked or unblocked. If one of your chakras was blocked, that meant that it wasn't working at all and there was something stopping it. Well, this is only half true. In fact, most of your chakras will work on some level since each one has a relationship—good or bad—to the facet of life it presides over and the body part it resides in. It's simply a matter of degree. Therefore, some chakras might be more active than others. As we discussed previously, this is the reason activation alone does not necessarily work perfectly, and why you need to balance them as well to make sure all the chakras are operating at the same frequency. If you don't balance, then your activation might result in you relying unevenly on one chakra or another. Balancing ensures that all the chakras are working just enough—not too hard and not too little—allowing each other to have an equal part in your overall health. After all, each chakra is important in its own way, functioning as part of a necessary whole.

How to Tell if Your Chakras Are Imbalanced

Back in Chapter 5 when we discussed individual chakras, we talked a little bit about how to tell when your chakras are blocked. Here, we will go a bit deeper and dive into how your chakras might look if they are overactive or underactive. Understanding why both of these things are negative is essential to the practice of balancing your chakras. In this section, we will first look at overall signs of imbalance then go into the individual chakras and outline some of the signs that the chakra is either overactive or underactive.

Overall Chakras

When your chakras are generally unbalanced, you will likely feel it in your body and your mind. Your health might be all over the place, being healthy one month but sick the next. You might also have uneven pains throughout your body. Psychologically, you might feel like you have a very skewed sense of self-esteem, perhaps being extremely confident in some areas but very shy in others. You might also struggle with relationships, being able to open up to people in some circumstances but not others, or struggling to connect on every level with a partner. This can cause frustration for yourself and others. Finally, you will likely feel spiritually disconnected, unable to truly transcend the everyday and think about those big spiritual questions with any clarity. These symptoms often mean that you have overactive and underactive chakras, leading your body to be severely unbalanced.

Root

When your root chakra is unbalanced, you will feel unrooted in some way; however, the way you feel this and how it manifests will look different depending on whether your root chakra is over- or underactive.

Overactive

An overactive root chakra looks like survival mode. You will feel like you need to greatly overcompensate for your feelings of uprootedness and insecurity. This might lead to an insecure attachment style or very conscious feelings of lostness.

Underactive

If your root chakra is underactive, on the other hand, this will likely manifest slightly differently, creating a more dreamy existence that isn't exactly aware of its lack of roots. You might tend to live in a fantasy world, not truly connected to those around you. It might not be as uncomfortable an existence as an overactive root chakra, but it will likely feel empty and as though it doesn't have much substance.

Sacral

Your sacral chakra's unbalanced symptoms will always affect your relationship to work versus pleasure. However, the side of the spectrum on which it falls will be greatly affected by whether your sacral chakra is over- or underactive.

Overactive

If your sacral chakra is overactive, then your appetite for pleasure will be insatiable. While this might sound like fun, it can end up manifesting as addictive behavior. Addiction to unhealthy food, alcohol, sex, or even dangerous drugs can follow from an overactive sacral chakra, which is completely focused on pleasure.

Underactive

When your sacral chakra is underactive, however, then you will most likely swing to the other side of the spectrum, depriving yourself of even the most harmless pleasures in life. This can lead to you becoming antisocial, prudish, depressed, and even impotent. Through excessive restriction, those with underactive sacral chakras end up with a stunted ability to experience pleasure in life.

Solar Plexus

Because the solar plexus chakra is related to self-esteem, the relative balance of that chakra will almost always manifest in the form of one's level of self-consciousness and feelings of power over others. As with the sacral chakra, the difference between an overactive and an underactive solar plexus chakra will put you on either end of the spectrum.

Overactive

If you have an overactive solar plexus chakra, then you will likely have a highly overinflated sense of self. You might feel superiority over other people and tend toward manipulative or controlling behavior. Those with overactive solar plexus chakras might be perceived as narcissistic by others, and they might even lack empathy and struggle to feel compassion for others.

Underactive

However, when this chakra is underactive, then there is a serious danger of becoming extremely low in confidence, ultimately struggling to have any sense of your own worth. These people will be the complete opposite of the narcissistic overactive chakra, becoming doormats or failing to speak up for themselves.

Heart

Your heart chakra's relative activity manifests itself through relationships. More specifically, it deals with your prioritization of needs and the way you manage boundaries. Where you fall on this spectrum will correspond to the relative over- or underactivity of your heart chakra.

Overactive

Those with overactive heart chakras will be very overeager in relationships and devote themselves entirely to their partner. Though this may sound like a good thing, it can have two distinct negative consequences, one for the individual and one for their loved one. For the individual, this often leads to a loss of self to the relationship, creating a sense that they are completely in that relationship and have no sense of autonomy anymore. For their loved one, this can result in added pressure and crossing of boundaries. A person with an overactive heart chakra might be hurt when loved ones set boundaries or take time for themselves, not understanding the concept of personal space.

Underactive

When someone's heart chakra is underactive, they will be very closed off to love. While they might not be outwardly cold or cruel to others, they might really struggle to let others in, meaning that their relationships struggle to progress past the initial stages. They might be afraid of the vulnerability that comes from loving someone or even of just pursuing someone and thus avoid relationships at all costs.

Throat

The throat chakra is all about voice. Not just your physical voice, but your metaphorical voice as well—how comfortable you feel expressing yourself and arguing your case in front of others. Your degree of confidence in your voice will ultimately be determined by the relative activity of your throat chakra.

Overactive

People with overactive throat chakras will appear similar to those with overactive solar plexus chakras. That is, they will seem overconfident and uninterested in others. However, for the person with an overactive throat chakra, it will manifest in the way they speak. They might tend to talk over others or interrupt often, while at the same time struggling to listen effectively. They might want to seem more intelligent than they really are, causing them to speak with authority on matters they don't really know much about or even outright lie to make themselves look better.

Underactive

On the other hand, those with underactive throat chakras will struggle to express themselves and lack faith in what they say. They might have a strong sense of self-esteem, perhaps coming from a well-balanced solar plexus chakra, but it will be very internal and not easily expressed to others.

Third Eye

The way relative activity manifests in your third eye chakra is through your sense of the world around you. This makes it somewhat similar to the root chakra in terms of its effect on your perception of reality.

Overactive

Having an overactive third eye chakra might not on the surface seem like a bad thing. After all, seeing ahead is good, right? But it can often lead to a kind of perception of reality similar to the underactive root chakra. Those with an overactive third eye chakra might tend to be disconnected from reality or life, seeing only the grander picture and forgetting to appreciate the little things or the earthly pleasures that make life worth living.

Underactive

If you have an underactive third eye chakra, you will be the opposite. Interestingly, most people actually have an underactive third eye chakra. It means that you have not yet come to realize the grander narrative of your life. It is very hard to have a well-balanced third eye chakra early in life as the narrative of your life starts to take shape later as you begin to gain more spiritual wisdom.

Crown

As we know, the crown chakra is associated with the highest realities and your relationship with your spiritual life. It is not something that can actually be over- or underactive. It is merely the summation of your other chakras. Thus, an unbalanced crown chakra is caused by imbalances in your other chakras. Balance all of your chakras equally, and you will unlock the key to a properly balanced crown chakra.

Chapter 13:
How to Rebalance Your Chakras

So, what do you do if your chakras become unbalanced? Well, there are certain techniques you can use to balance them. You already know how to unblock your chakras by using the techniques we discussed back in Chapter 11, but balancing can be trickier. Overactive chakras can especially be difficult to balance since most of them involve major blind spots that can be difficult to acknowledge. In this chapter, we will lead you through some essential techniques for creating balance and harmony among your chakras.

Are Your Chakras Overactive or Underactive?

The first step to balancing your chakras is to determine whether they are underactive or overactive. It might be hard to tell at first, especially if you are experiencing physical symptoms. Even for psychological issues, it might be difficult to determine what exactly your issues are in relation to a particular chakra. Use the diagnostic traits in the last chapter to really ascertain where you stand on the scale of underactive to overactive. This might take a fair amount of self-reflection, especially for those with overactive throat or solar plexus chakras, which tend to manifest as overconfidence. When you are determining this scale, you have to be willing to see the negative side of yourself and possibly confront some very ugly truths. If you are willing to do this, then you will be able to successfully place yourself on the scale of underactive to overactive.

Chakra by Chakra

Now, the process of actually balancing your chakras is slightly different from the process of activation. When it comes to activation, it's all about connecting with each chakra. However, unbalanced chakras tend to be the result of an unmet need somewhere in your life. The unbalanced chakra is either responding to a deficiency by shutting down or overcompensating. In this sense, underactive and overactive chakras are two sides of the same coin; it just might take longer for those with overactive chakras to accept that they have a problem. Thus, the answer to balancing your chakras properly is to feed that unmet need it is responding to. Here, we will go chakra by chakra, explaining the core need that must be met in order for that chakra to be balanced properly.

Root

An imbalance in your root chakra is almost always a response to a sense of rootlessness in your real life. Maybe you've been moving around a lot lately or don't really have a permanent home. Maybe you just exited a long-term relationship and are struggling to redefine your identity independent of that person. Or maybe you are recently retired and don't know what your new life is going to look like. Consistent uncertainty and major changes in life will often manifest through an imbalance in the root chakra. To balance, try to anchor yourself to something concrete. Find something important to you that isn't changing and try to concentrate on it during your meditation practice. This will help you to create a context in which you feel safe without having to change your circumstances permanently.

Sacral

Over- or underactive sacral chakras are usually a response to a lack of constructive or fulfilling pleasure. Both people who abstain from and overdose on pleasure do not have a healthy relationship with it. Those who tend toward addiction struggle to find pleasure that fulfills them in a lasting way. They are always searching for their next "fix" because they lack truly fulfilling pleasure. Similarly, those who abstain from pleasure probably have a hard time connecting to pleasurable activities and are bogged down by shame. In both cases, you need to find an activity that is pleasurable in a more lasting way. Higher quality "junk food" such as cookies from an artisanal French bakery might help you get your sugar fix while also learning something about another culture and expanding your palate. If you're a TV junkie, try putting on a show you've never seen before or an interesting film. It's the same action, but you are expanding your mind at the same time. For both over- and underactive sacral chakras, you need to learn to appreciate "higher" pleasures or pleasures that expand your mind and yourself, leading to a more lasting feeling of fulfillment.

Solar Plexus

Because over- and underactive solar plexus chakras often manifest in terms of your levels of insecurity, you need to find ways to boost your confidence. Even though they might not seem like it, those with overactive solar plexus chakras can often be just as insecure as those with underactive ones. Their excessive boasting is often a kind of overcompensation wherein they feel the need to constantly project their greatness into the world. If you fall into either of these categories, you need to face your insecurities. Try to have a vulnerable moment with a friend where you are neither bragging nor holding back—simply show yourself in an honest light. Or, you can try to face some of your fears: speak in public, meet a new person, fly on an airplane. Any of these things will help you build a strong sense of inner confidence that does not rely on bragging for its foundation.

Heart

People with both over- and underactive heart chakras often have what's called an "insecure attachment style." An insecure attachment style is a method of connecting to other people wherein you never feel truly secure in your relationship with them. You might constantly fear that your loved ones are going to leave you, even if they have given no indication that they are going to do so. Interestingly, the main symptoms of an insecure attachment style include both the signs of an overactive heart chakra (excessive clinginess, lack of boundaries) and an underactive heart chakra (social withdrawal, fear of intimacy). Clearly, we can see that there is a connection and that your heart chakra being over- versus underactive are two sides of the same coin. To help combat both of these reactions, you need to build a stronger faith in the people around you. Remind yourself that they are there for you and that they will love you even if you make mistakes. Maybe even reach out to one of these people and let them know about the insecurity that you have. Even if you are someone who seeks reassurance often and your loved one is sick of giving it, approaching this in a more honest way and framing it around your own self-reflection will help them to give you more meaningful reassurance of their commitment to you. You should also remind yourself of your commitment to others. Often an unbalanced heart chakra, especially an underactive one, can result in fear of commitment since you are afraid of getting hurt. Therefore, reinforcing your own commitment to others is just as important as being reassured of their commitment to you.

Throat

Both overactive and underactive throat chakras are a direct response to a misuse of the voice. A lack of true confidence in your voice or a lack of interest in others' voices will usually be the cause of your overactive or underactive throat chakra. The solution, then, is to work on your communication skills, both input and output. For output, try to isolate the cause of your difficulty speaking. Do you tend to speak over people because you are afraid of not being heard? Are you reluctant to speak up because you are afraid you have nothing interesting to say? One good exercise is to engage in some reflective writing. This allows you to use your "voice" outside the presence of other people. Write about something you're interested in and notice how you feel differently when you are writing versus speaking. For input, you need to do some exercises to improve your listening skills, both as a model for how you should be speaking and to help you listen better to other people. Put on some podcasts and try to be a really active listener. Note what the people are saying and truly take in their information. Then, write another reflective piece about what you liked about their words and how they said them. Reinforcing the two-way nature of communication will help you achieve more balance within your throat chakra.

Third Eye

The main cause of an unbalanced third eye chakra, whether it is manifesting as overactive or underactive, is a lack of connection between your spiritual life and your everyday life. Those with overactive third eye chakras tend to overlook the little everyday things in life, and those with underactive third eye chakras tend to miss the spiritual world. Both of these outcomes are negative since you lack the connection that allows you to live a more spiritually connected life. The best way to help balance your third eye chakra is to practice mindfulness. Mindfulness is the perfect remedy to an unbalanced third eye chakra because it endeavors to do just what you need: connect the spiritual and everyday realms. Noticing the unique tranquility or beauty of a leaf or a butterfly can do wonders for making the everyday spiritual and the spiritual everyday. By cultivating a strong mindfulness practice, you will be able to effectively balance your third eye chakra and create a stronger connection between your spiritual and physical self.

Pillar 6: Healing

The third major way people interact with their chakras is through healing. Healing your chakras is an ancient practice and happens when people feel like their chakras are blocked or severely unbalanced. You can even experience chakra trauma which can lead to terrible repercussions for the rest of your body. In this pillar, we will be exploring some of the ways in which people specifically use healing practices to help their chakras. First, we will be discussing five different specific healing traditions: Ayurveda, yoga, meditation, psychotherapy, and Reiki. Through these five techniques, you will learn some alternative ways you can interact with your chakras. Then, we will talk about different areas of your life in which chakra healing can have a powerful effect. By the end of this section, you should know how to heal your chakras and what that healing can be used for.

Chapter 14: Practices

There are many different ways to interact with your chakras. We've already talked about a few of them in the last two pillars when we shared techniques for activation and balancing. But here, we are going to talk about some of the methods that are commonly used in healing specifically. These practices range from ancient to modern and cover a wide range of different chakra needs. Selecting a method will depend on a number of factors, including the chakra you are needing to heal, the depth of your trauma, and how you want to go about healing as well as your involvement with other spiritual practices. In this chapter, we will explore five of these methods so that you can construct your own version of chakra healing that incorporates the best of all worlds. At the end of this chapter, you should have a solid understanding of these techniques and a good idea of which ones might be most beneficial to you.

Ayurveda

A system of medicine that runs adjacent to and is often associated with chakras is Ayurveda. It originated in ancient South Asia, just like the chakras. You will probably notice the word "Veda" as part of Ayurveda, which is no coincidence since it is also derived from the same texts as chakras. However, this medicinal practice focuses on holistic healing that incorporates aspects like diet, exercise, psychology, and spirituality, among other things. This approach to medicine is often adopted in the West as a response to the relatively single-minded approaches in Western medicine. With Ayurvedic medicine, you will be able to treat and check in with the whole body. Similar to chakras, it acknowledges that the body is a system, not just a series of unrelated organs, and thus is aware that the process of healing will always involve more than one healing practice. When you engage with Ayurvedic medicine, you will not be able to heal one area of the body without checking in on all the others, which helps to bring a more holistic awareness to the body.

The Four Pillars of Ayurveda

There are actually four main pillars of Ayurveda healing that can be used to help your body. In this section, we will give you an overview of these four pillars.

1. *Tridosha*

    The Tridosha are the three basic bioenergies that circulate through your body. These energies regulate all of your body's functions, helping you to stay alive and healthy.

2. *Triguna*

    The Triguna are the three basic properties of the universe. These consist of the pure, the dynamic, and the inert. They circulate through both our bodies and space to bring connections throughout the world.

3. Five Mahabhutas

The five Mahabhutas are actually something we've already discussed. These are the five basic elements of the world: earth, water, air, fire, and ether.

4. Chorashi Ousodhi

Finally, the Chorashi Ousodhi are the 84 herbs that are central to Ayurveda healing. These herbs are incredibly important and will be vital to our discussion of Ayurveda and the chakras.

Ayurveda and Chakras

So, how do you use this medicine alongside chakras? Well, we have already discussed some of the other aspects of Ayurvedic healing in tandem with the chakras, so in this section, we will focus on the herbs associated with each chakra. This is a fascinating way that we can see the connection between what we put in our bodies and how we feel. These herbs or foods can target specific chakras and help to heal them through the supplementation of necessary nutrients. In this section, we will list the seven chakras alongside the Ayurvedic recommendations for foods or herbs to add to your diet.

Root

For your root chakra, the Ayurvedic texts recommend, unsurprisingly, root vegetables. These will help you quite literally connect with your roots and with the earth. These vegetables often contain traces of dirt or organic matter which can actually be quite healthy to ingest in small doses. This organic matter contains microbes that can do wonders for your guts. Try incorporating more vegetables like carrots, beets, and even potatoes into your diet to help your root chakra heal and grow.

Sacral

For the sacral chakra, you want to eat things that are beneficial to your digestive tract. These are usually anti-inflammatory or gut health-promoting herbs or foods that can do wonders for your sacral chakra's function. There is also a lot of evidence that the way you treat your gut has strong implications for your mental health. Thus, even the psychological aspects of your sacral chakra can be healed through your gut. In general, fermented foods such as kombucha, kimchi, or sauerkraut can be great ways to heal and repair your gut. Two other important herbs have been mentioned in Vedic texts in relation to the sacral chakra for centuries: nagarmotha and gurmar. These are both easy-to-find plants that will do wonders if you are experiencing blocks with your sacral chakra.

Solar Plexus

For your solar plexus chakra, you want to eat things that target your digestive tract as well, but more in the stomach rather than the gut territory. Thus, you want to focus more intensely on anti-inflammatory spices. Cardamom and fenugreek are two of the best herbs to keep your stomach calm and facilitate healthy digestion.

Heart

For your heart chakra, you want to eat for cardiovascular health. Fiber and iron are two very important nutrients to help with your heart and blood systems. From the Ayurveda perspective, garcinia and sandalwood oil are two of the most important herbs to take if you are experiencing a blocked heart chakra.

Throat

For your throat, you want to focus on things that are going to prevent the most common illness associated with a blocked throat chakra: sinus infections. Foods with a high vitamin C content are great, especially fruits like berries and citrus. According to Ayurveda, you should also be taking things that are clarifying since clarity and honesty are traits associated with a well-balanced throat chakra. Thus, sage and guggulu are some of the best ones to take to help balance out and promote health within your throat chakra.

Third Eye

Your third eye chakra needs brain-nourishing food as well as food that promotes clarity of thought and a sound balance between your mind and body. For this, one of the best things recommended by Ayurveda is ginkgo biloba, which helps you to gain that clarity of sight so central to the third eye chakra.

Crown

For your crown chakra, you want to be awakening your highest forms of thinking and self. For this, you should be promoting beauty in your life. This is why Ayurveda promotes lavender as the herb of choice. You can bring lavender into your life in the form of tea, edible lavender, or even burning lavender incense or candles in your space to form that close connection.

Yoga

One practice that we haven't talked about too much directly throughout this book is yoga. We have addressed it peripherally, but it is really one of the most important chakra-adjacent practices. Yoga is incredibly important to your chakra healing journey because it is all about opening up the body. With yoga, you are moving your body in ways you never thought possible, using muscles and stretching joints you didn't even know you had. By engaging in the practice of yoga, you are helping to build better awareness of your body and creating a connection to your chakras. Here, we will list for you some of the best yoga poses for healing each of your chakras.

Root

To heal your root chakra, you should try poses that help to ground you in the earth. Mountain pose and warrior pose are the best for this since they help you with balance and energy flow between your body and the ground below it.

Sacral

One of the leading causes of digestive issues is lack of exercise and movement in the core. For this reason, expanding and compressing your abdomen is especially helpful for the sacral chakra. Forward bends, either standing or sitting, are some of the best ways to release tension within your sacral chakra and help build a better core.

Solar Plexus

The solar plexus is connected with the element of the sun, hence the name. Thus, yoga sun salutation sequences are strongly associated with the solar plexus chakra. Performing a whole sun salutation every day, or at least often, will help you connect with your solar plexus chakra and start your journey toward healing it.

Heart

For your heart, it's all about opening up your chest. Back in Chapter 13, we talked about how embracing vulnerability and opening yourself up to the world is essential for the heart chakra, so you really need to build this into your yoga practice. Cobra pose is a great one because it lifts the chest to the sky, exposing it, stretching it, and elevating it at the same time. Practicing poses like this will build strength in your heart chakra.

Throat

As with the heart, we want to expose this chakra to the world to help banish insecurity and negative thoughts. Cat pose, where you alternately round and arch your back, can help you to really get that flow moving in your neck, creating a sense of positive vulnerability that can help you start getting over some of your communication-based fears.

Third Eye

The third eye chakra is all about gaining a certain perspective on the world. Since our eyes are always at the top of our bodies, it can be good to reverse this by going into child's pose. In this pose, your forehead is on the ground, helping to build that connection between your third eye and the earth.

Meditation

Along the same lines as yoga, we have meditation. Again, we have already brought up meditation periodically throughout this book. When it comes to meditating with your chakras, it's all about connecting that certain facet of life with that certain part of your body. Sometimes, we feel disconnected from our bodies, so focusing on them can help you to find solutions to problems that you never would have thought of otherwise. It can also help you to feel more validated in some of your concerns. If you have had chronic anxiety your entire life but don't know why, it's very useful to be able to point to something concrete that is causing it and have multiple techniques ready so you can work on that anxiety going forward. Thus, meditating with your chakras brings awareness to your meditation practice and to your body as a whole.

Psychotherapy

Some people, especially those who have already been to therapy or are currently in therapy, find it useful to incorporate chakra healing into the process. Looking at your issues through the lens of chakra imbalances can help put some of your thoughts and feelings into words. You might be able to pinpoint certain times in your life, even traumatic incidents, wherein you felt like your chakras might have been thrown out of balance for whatever reason, preventing you from living your life to the fullest. It can help certain psychiatric practices take shape, especially in the form of creating a narrative. However, because of the medical nature of many psychiatry degrees, not all psychiatrists will take chakra healing seriously. If you are serious about chakra healing, you will either want to find a psychotherapist who specializes in chakra healing or at least is open to it as an aspect of your therapeutic journey. After all, there's nothing worse than being dismissed by the person who is meant to help you!

Reiki

Finally, you can use Reiki, a Japanese form of energy healing that can do wonders for your mind and body, especially when used in tandem with your chakras. This practice involves a Reiki healer using their energies to help you promote your own. It is based on a very similar ideology to that of chakras, and thus the two practices can be used in tandem with one another for maximum effect. Find a Reiki healer to help you promote your healing journey. Many healers can be found in most major towns and cities, so consider trying it out to ensure that you are maximizing all resources in relation to energy healing.

Chapter 15:
Remedies

Almost everyone has gone through some kind of hardship in their life. And for a lot of people, these struggles can be ongoing. You might suffer from a particular ailment, be it physical or psychological, for many years. If you don't have the tools to help yourself heal from these things, they can seem very scary. Throughout this book, we have listed a number of solutions to many problems that a lot of people face in their lives. In this chapter, we will go more in-depth about each of these ailments that can be helped through chakra healing. You can think of this section as being a kind of index to help you keep track of all the things you can do with the power of chakras. By the end of this chapter, you should have a firm grasp on all the amazing things chakras can do to help you!

Allergies

Seasonal allergies can be a nuisance, but did you know that chakra healing can actually do a lot to alleviate them? This ailment is most often associated with an unbalanced or traumatized heart chakra. Because allergies are related to an overactive immune system, it can often actually be an overactive heart chakra that can be at the root of the issue. By healing your heart chakra, you might be able to relieve your allergies.

Anger Management

Who among us hasn't gotten angry before in their lives? Sometimes anger can be healthy, fueling your sense of justice or self-worth. However, anger can just as often be unhealthy. Some people might even find that they struggle with chronic anger management issues. Fortunately, chakra healing might actually be able to help you with this. Oftentimes, anger stems from deep feelings of being underappreciated or unloved. Thus, the heart chakra and solar plexus chakras—the ones most responsible for your relationships with others—might be blocked if you are experiencing chronic uncontrollable anger. Consider healing these chakras in order to get a better hold on your anger.

Anxiety

Generalized anxiety is one of the most common issues people experience. Especially in a world as chaotic as ours, it's almost impossible not to feel anxious all the time. Chakra healing can do wonders for anxiety. However, since anxiety is so general, almost all chakras have a part to play. Doing some inner work, either alone or with a therapist, can help you trace the specific type of anxiety you happen to be experiencing and thus pinpoint the specific chakra you should be targeting to help it.

Back Pain

Related to anxiety, and therefore to the chakras, is back pain. Because the back is long, it actually connects to all the chakras as well. The spinal cord, which covers your entire back, is said to be the central point of all the chakras. As with anxiety, it is useful to pinpoint where on your back you are experiencing pain in order to identify the correct chakra to heal.

Codependency

It's healthy to depend on other people and have others depend on you. After all, that's what friend circles and family units are for. However, there is a type of dependency that can become unhealthy. This is when someone relies on someone else to an unhealthy degree, perhaps even preventing that other person from being happy in order to stay connected to them. If you are struggling with codependency, then you likely also have an imbalance in your heart chakra—probably overactive. Setting boundaries and balancing out your heart chakra will help you to create healthy relationships with proper distance.

Confidence

Confidence is a topic we have talked about fairly extensively throughout this book. Generally, confidence is like anxiety and can be connected to many of the chakras. However, the lower ones, especially root and sacral, will contain the deepest confidence issues. If you struggle with chronic low self-esteem, it would be best to start with these lower chakras to target those deeper insecurities and then gradually work your way up the chakra system.

Headaches

Migraines or chronic headaches are also common problems for many people. They can be caused by a variety of things ranging from poor gut health to iron deficiencies to eye strain. Thus, a complete balancing of all of your chakras is needed in order to help ameliorate headache issues you might be experiencing. That being said, you might also want to check specifically on your third eye chakra since this tends to be the chakra most associated with headaches.

Joints

Many people also suffer from joint pain. We in the West live very sedentary lifestyles, often with sedentary jobs and hobbies. Sitting too much and not incorporating proper stretching techniques into your everyday life can have devastating consequences on your physical and mental health. Chakra healing, especially if it is combined with yoga practice, can help you to open up some of those joints and build flexibility and bring flow back into your body.

Sex

Even though it remains a taboo topic in many parts of the world, sexual issues are all too common. Whether it's addiction or repression, many people struggle to maintain a healthy relationship with their sexuality. The first step in this process is to focus on your sacral chakra, which is the sexual center of your body, among other things. If you are having sexual issues with a long-term partner, you might also want to check in with your heart chakra to make sure you are providing enough care to one another as well as with your throat chakra to ensure that you are communicating properly. At the end of the day, self-esteem and communication skills are the backbone of a healthy sex life.

Trauma

Finally, it's an unfortunate fact that many people have experienced trauma in their lives. Incidents such as deaths, assaults, or even dramatic moves can cause a person to become traumatized for life. Oftentimes, we hold this trauma in our bodies as well as our minds, which makes chakra healing perfect as a trauma healer. Identifying the source of your trauma will help you to determine which chakra you need to address in order for you to start to heal.

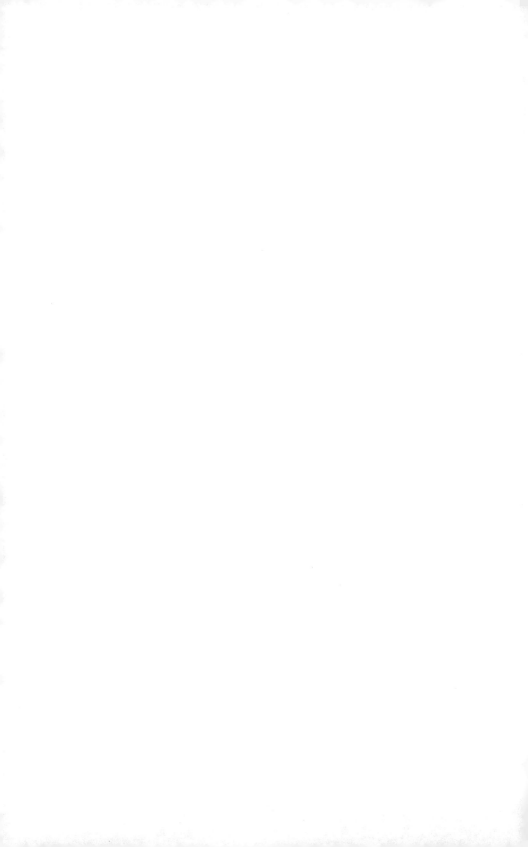

Conclusion

The chakras are a complex system. They consist of many different systems, coincide with countless other spiritual practices, and account for a multitude of functions throughout your body. However, if understood properly, they can be a great asset for your happiness and your health. Throughout this book, we have endeavored to enlighten you on some of the most essential aspects of the chakra healing process. We have led you through all the essential aspects of chakra healing, helping you to see how chakras work. We have detailed the history of the chakras, showing you where they came from and the cultural context in which they evolved. Then, we discussed each of the chakras in isolation and discussed the aspects of life as well as body parts over which each of the chakras presides. Moving forward, we talked about ways you can manage your chakras, either through activation, balancing, or healing. Through all of this, you have gained priceless knowledge about the chakras and the place they can have in your life. You now have the tools to get out there and start healing your chakras!

If you learned from this book, we would really appreciate seeing a review from you. We take a lot of pride in our books and would love to hear what our readers think. Building community and sharing your experience is what spiritual learning and healing are all about. We ensure that our books inform people about things that can help them in their real lives. After reading this book, you are now equipped with the knowledge of one of the most powerful and ancient systems in the world, leading you toward a path of enlightenment and health. Chakra healing isn't for the faint of heart—it's for the ones who really want to dig deep into their innermost selves and heal themselves in ways they didn't know were possible. It might be a long journey ahead, but you are now prepared to go out and do it for yourself. So, go out into the world and get healing!

Glossary

Astrology: A spiritual system based on the positions of stars and planets. Conventionally, it consists of 12 zodiac signs, 7 planets, and 12 houses.

Ayurveda: A type of Vedic healing that focuses on holistic practice, including diet and spirituality.

Blocked chakra: A chakra through which energy is not flowing properly.

Buddhism: A religion that started in Northern India in the 4th century B.C.E.

Chakra: A point on your body that consists of a specific kind of energy. Originating from the Vedic text of Ancient South Asia.

Chakra activation: Helping your chakras to open and work to their full potential.

Chakra balancing: Making sure your chakras are operating at the right frequency relative to one another.

Chakra healing: Bringing your chakras back to proper health.

Chorashi Ousodhi: The 84 herbs that form the foundation of Ayurvedic healing.

Crown chakra: The highest chakra on the body, located at the top of the head. Associated with the highest forms of spiritual learning.

Crystal healing: A spiritual practice that uses the natural vibrations of crystals to heal the body.

Divine chakra: The fifth and highest of the higher chakras, located in infinite space and associated with divine knowledge.

Earth star chakra: The first of the higher chakras located a foot below the feet, associated with the spiritual knowledge of the earth.

Endocrine system: A medical system that connects some of the major organs and glands of the body and which can easily be mapped onto the chakra system.

Five Mahabhutas: The five elements as represented in the Ayurveda system.

Galactic chakra: The fourth chakra in the higher chakra system, located two feet above the head.

Heart chakra: The fourth chakra located in the chest, associated with love and relationships.

Hinduism: An ancient but currently practiced religion developed thousands of years ago in South Asia.

Ida nadi: The nadi on the left side of the body associated with femininity.

Nadi: A parallel chakra system that runs from the left to the right of the body.

Overactive chakra: A chakra that has overcompensated, resulting in exaggerated, often negative versions of that chakra.

Pingala nadi: The nadi on the right side of the body associated with masculinity.

Prana: The chakra word for energy.

Reiki: A type of healing that involves transferring energy through the hands.

Root chakra: The first chakra located at the bottom of the spine, associated with groundedness and stability.

Sacral chakra: The second chakra located in the lower abdomen, associated with intimacy and creativity.

Solar plexus chakra: The third chakra located in the stomach, associated with self-esteem and socializing.

Soul star chakra: The second chakra in the higher chakra system, located six inches above the top of the head.

Sushumna nadi: The center nadi located in the center of the spine, associated with the balance between the ida and pingala nadi.

Tarot: A spiritual system of cards that can be used for divination or self-discovery.

Third eye chakra: The sixth chakra located between the eyes, associated with foresight and wisdom.

Throat chakra: The fifth chakra located in the throat, associated with communication and honesty.

Underactive chakra: A chakra that is operating at a lower frequency in comparison to the others.

Universal chakra: The third chakra in the higher chakra system.

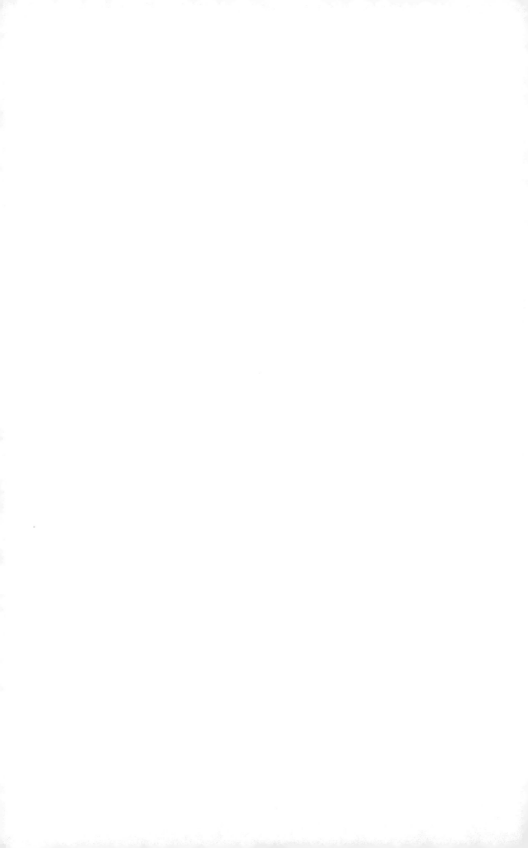

References

Anatomy of the endocrine system. (2019). Johns Hopkins Medicine. https://www.hopkinsmedicine.org/health/wellness-and-prevention/anatomy-of-the-endocrine-system

Ayurveda. (2019, December 2). Hopkins Medicine. https://www.hopkinsmedicine.org/health/wellness-and-prevention/ayurveda#:~:text=What%20is%20Ayurveda%3F

Balanced chakras reduce anxiety. (n.d.). Anxiety. https://www.anxiety.org/balance-your-chakras-let-your-anxiety-melt-away

Burney, R. (2017, January 21). *Chakra levels of consciousness.* Codependency Recovery. https://codependentrecoveryexpert.wordpress.com/2017/01/21/chakra-levels-of-consciousness/

Chakra | religion. (n.d.). Encyclopedia Britannica. https://www.britannica.com/topic/chakra

Chakra elements and their meanings. (n.d.). 7 Chakra Store. https://7chakrastore.com/blogs/news/chakra-elements

Chakra endocrine system | PDF | thyroid | adrenal gland. (n.d.). Scribd. https://www.scribd.com/document/200345709/Chakra-Endocrine-System

Chakra yoga explained—A full guide to the 7 chakras. (n.d.). TINT Yoga. https://tintyoga.com/magazine/chakra-yoga/

Chakras and Buddhism. (2019, August 15). The Zen Universe. https://thezenuniverse.org/chakras-and-buddhism-the-zen-universe/

Chakras, colors & Hindu gods: A closer look at the Hindu system. (n.d.). Lotus Sculpture. https://www.lotussculpture.com/blog/chakras-colors-hindu-gods/

Chakras: A beginner's guide to the 7 chakras. (2016, October 4). Healthline. https://www.healthline.com/health/fitness-exercise/7-chakras#Chakra-101

Complete guide to the 7 chakras: Symbols, effects & how to balance. (2019, June 13). Arhanta Yoga Blog. https://www.arhantayoga.org/blog/7-chakras-introduction-energy-centers-effect/#:~:text=Symptoms%20and%20Effects-

Doniger, W. (2019). *Ganesha | meaning, symbolism, & facts.* Encyclopædia Britannica. https://www.britannica.com/topic/Ganesha

Earth star chakra: What it is & why it matters. (2022, April 12). Be My Travel Muse. https://www.bemytravelmuse.com/earth-star-chakra/

Element of air in tarot cards. (n.d.). Corax. https://www.corax.com/tarot/element-of-air.html

Element of earth in tarot cards. (n.d.). Corax. https://www.corax.com/tarot/element-of-earth.html

Element of fire in tarot cards. (n.d.). Corax. https://www.corax.com/tarot/element-of-fire.html

Element of water in tarot cards. (n.d.). Corax. https://www.corax.com/tarot/element-of-water.html

Feeling out of sorts? Here's how to balance your chakras. (2020, January 4). Well+Good. https://www.wellandgood.com/chakra-balancing/

Fire element crystals: 9 best healing stones to balance your elements. (2021, November 14). Crystals Alchemy. https://crystalsalchemy.com/fire-element-crystals

5 common misconceptions about chakras. (2018, October 1). Himalayan Institute Online. https://himalayaninstitute.org/online/5-common-misconceptions-chakras/

5 ways to heal your knee chakras. (2012, September 12). Mindbodygreen. https://www.mindbodygreen.com/articles/how-to-heal-your-knee-chakras

The genital or pubic chakra. (n.d.). Malankazlev. http://malankazlev.com/kheper/topics/chakras/Pubic.htm

Get to know the seven chakras. (n.d.). Yoloha Yoga. https://yolohayoga.com/en-ca/blogs/yoloha-life/get-to-know-the-seven-chakras#:~:text=A%20person%20with%20an%20overactive

Hindu deity Vishnu. (n.d.). Khan Academy. https://www.khanacademy.org/humanities/art-asia/beginners-guide-asian-culture/hindu-art-culture/a/hindu-deity-vishnu#:~:text=Vishnu%20is%20the%20god%20of

How attachment styles affect adult relationships. (n.d.). Helpguide. https://www.helpguide.org/articles/relationships-communication/attachment-and-adult-relationships.htm#:~:text=Attachment%20styles%20and%20how%20they%20shape%20adult%20relationships&text=Those%20with%20insecure%20attachment%20styles

How do you know if your chakras are open? (2020, May 12). Beadnova. https://www.beadnova.com/blog/12981/how-do-you-know-if-your-chakra-is-open-or-blocked

How to activate chakras in your body? (2021, February 4). Best Wellness Resort. https://www.dharanaretreat.com/blogs/how-to-activate-chakras-in-your-body/#:~:text=Sit%20on%20your%20knees%2C%20with

How to identify & heal blocked chakras. (2019, January 27). Mindvalley Blog. https://blog.mindvalley.com/symptoms-of-blocked-chakras/

Hueneburg, K. (2021, October 19). *The complete guide to understanding the chakras.* One Yoga. https://oneyogathailand.com/the-complete-guide-to-understanding-the-chakras/

Importance of foot chakra. (2015, May 1). Reiki Rays. https://reikirays.com/21123/importance-of-foot-chakra/

Jackson, D. (2020a, August 18). *Higher chakras series: Exploring the universal chakra.* AskAstrology. https://askastrology.com/universal-chakra/

Jackson, D. (2020b, August 29). *Higher chakras series: Exploring the galactic chakra.* AskAstrology. https://askastrology.com/galactic-chakra/

Jackson, D. (2020c, September 4). *Higher chakras series: Exploring the divine gateway chakra*. AskAstrology. https://askastrology.com/divine-gateway-chakra/

Learn about your seven chakras and how to keep them in balance. (2020, January 8). Chopra. https://chopra.com/articles/learn-about-your-seven-chakras-and-how-to-keep-them-in-balance

Mughal dynasty | history, map, & facts. (2018). Encyclopædia Britannica. https://www.britannica.com/topic/Mughal-dynasty

9 powerful air element crystals for inspiration. (2021, November 15). Crystals Alchemy. https://crystalsalchemy.com/air-element-crystals

9 powerful water element crystals for love and inner peace. (2021, November 17). Crystals Alchemy. https://crystalsalchemy.com/water-element-crystals

Peters, J. (2021, August 3). *Exploring the spiritual meaning of lower back pain*. Spirituality & Health. https://www.spiritualityhealth.com/exploring-the-spiritual-meaning-of-lower-back-pain

Planets and chakras. (n.d.). Sahaja Yoga Portal. https://www.sahajayogaportal.org/en/astrology/planets-chakras.html#:~:text=Chakras%20display%20the%20nature%20and

A primer of the chakra system. (2020, August 20). Chopra. https://chopra.com/articles/what-is-a-chakra#:~:text=The%20chakra%20system%20holds%20your

Raveesh, B. (2013). Ardhanareeshwara concept: Brain and psychiatry. *Indian Journal of Psychiatry, 55*(6), 263. https://doi.org/10.4103/0019-5545.105548

Ray, D. A. (2021, February 20). *Ayurveda and the 7 chakras: A step by step guide*. Amit Ray. https://amitray.com/ayurveda-and-the-7-chakras-a-beginners-guide/

7 chakras in human body, significance & how to balance them. (n.d.). Art of Living (India). https://www.artofliving.org/in-en/meditation/meditation-benefits/seven-chakras-explained

Seven crystals associated with the earth element. (n.d.). Exemplore. https://exemplore.com/healing/Seven-Crystals-Associated-with-the-Earth-Element

Symptoms of allergies, how to cure and get treatment of allergies. (n.d.). Rudraksha Ratna. https://www.rudraksha-ratna.com/articles/allergies

Tantrik studies. (2016, February 6). Tantrik Studies. https://hareesh.org/blog/2016/2/5/the-real-story-on-the-chakras

Vail, L. F. (2018). *The origins of Buddhism*. Asia Society. https://asiasociety.org/education/origins-buddhism

van der Kolk, B. (2014, September 25). *The body keeps the score: Brain, mind, and body in the healing of trauma*. Viking Press.

What are nadis? Your guide to energy channels in your body. (2021, April 19). Brett Larkin Yoga. https://www.brettlarkin.com/nadis-in-yoga/

What is ida nadi? (n.d.). Yogapedia. https://www.yogapedia.com/definition/5374/ida-nadi

What is ishvara? (n.d.). Yogapedia. https://www.yogapedia.com/definition/5296/ishvara

What is nadi? (n.d.). Yogapedia. https://www.yogapedia.com/definition/5028/nadi

What is sadashiva? (n.d.). Yogapedia. https://www.yogapedia.com/definition/7680/sadashiva

What is the origin of the chakra system? (n.d.). Indigo Massage & Wellness. https://indigomassagetherapy.com/uncategorized/what-is-the-origin-of-the-chakra-system/#:~:text=The%20chakra%20system%20originated%20in

What is the soul star chakra and how to connect to it. (n.d.). Zennedout. https://zennedout.com/what-is-the-soul-star-chakra-and-how-to-connect-to-it/

Where did Buddhism originate? (n.d.). History Hit. https://www.historyhit.com/where-did-buddhism-originate/

Why Lord Shiva is the most fascinating Hindu deity. (2009). Learn Religions. https://www.learnreligions.com/lord-shiva-basics-1770459

Willis, K. K. (2016, January 18). *Grief and rage: The connection between 4th and 1st chakras*. Lucid Body. https://lucidbody.com/blog/grief-and-rage-the-connection-between-4th-and

Made in the USA
Coppell, TX
01 April 2024

30762160R10085